Root Cause Analysis in Health Care

Tools and Techniques

THIRD EDITION

Senior Editor: Jennie McKee
Project Manager: Jan Kendrick
Manager, Publications: Eileen Norris
Production Manager: Johanna Harris
Associate Director: Cecily Pew
Executive Director: Catherine Chopp Hinckley
Vice President, Learning: George J. Farina
Joint Commission/JCR Reviewers: Rick Croteau, Coleen McKenna, Robert Katzfey, Celeste Milton, Judy Homa-Lowry, Cherie Ulaskas, Eileen Norris, Cecily Pew

Joint Commission Resources Mission

The mission of Joint Commission Resources is to continuously improve the safety and quality of care in the United States and in the international community through the provision of education and consultation services and international accreditation.

Joint Commission Resources educational programs and publications support, but are separate from, the accreditation activities of the Joint Commission. Attendees at Joint Commission Resources educational programs and purchasers of Joint Commission Resources publications receive no special consideration or treatment in, or confidential information about, the accreditation process.

The inclusion of an organization name, product, or service in a Joint Commission publication should not be construed as an endorsement of such organization, product, or services, nor is failure to include an organization name, product, or service to be construed as disapproval.

This publication is designed to provide accurate and authoritative information in regard to the subject matter covered. Every attempt has been made to ensure accuracy at the time of publication; however, please note that laws, regulations, and standards are subject to change. Please also note that some of the examples in this publication are specific to the laws and regulations of the locality of the facility. The information and examples in this publication are provided with the understanding that the publisher is not engaged in providing medical, legal, or other professional advice. If any such assistance is desired, the services of a competent professional person should be sought.

© 2005 by the Joint Commission on Accreditation of Healthcare Organizations

Joint Commission Resources, Inc. (JCR), a not-for-profit affiliate of the Joint Commission on Accreditation of Healthcare Organizations (Joint Commission), has been designated by the Joint Commission to publish publications and multimedia products. JCR reproduces and distributes these materials under license from the Joint Commission.

All rights reserved. No part of this publication may be reproduced in any form or by any means without written permission from the publisher.

Printed in the U.S.A. 5 4 3 2 1

Requests for permission to make copies of any part of this work should be mailed to
Permissions Editor
Department of Publications
Joint Commission Resources
One Renaissance Boulevard
Oakbrook Terrace, Illinois 60181
permissions@jcrinc.com

ISBN: 0-86688-909-4
ISSN: OR Library of Congress Control Number: 2005925230

For more information about Joint Commission Resources, please visit http://www.jcrinc.com.

Table of Contents

Introduction 1

Chapter 1. Root Cause Analysis: An Overview 7
    What Is Root Cause Analysis? 7
    When Can a Root Cause Analysis Be Performed? 7
    Variation and the Difference Between Proximate and Root Causes 8
    Benefits of Root Cause Analysis 10
    The Root Cause Analysis and Action Plan: Doing It Right 14

Chapter 2. Developing and Implementing a Policy and an Early Response Strategy for Sentinel Events 25
    Sentinel Events and the Range of Adverse Events in Health Care 25
    Leadership, Culture, and Sentinel Events 26
    The Joint Commission's Sentinel Event Policy 27
    Developing a Sentinel Event Policy 38
    Early Response Strategies 40
    Event Investigation 40
    Onward with Root Cause Analysis 47

Chapter 3. Preparing for Root Cause Analysis 49
    Step One: Organize a Team 49
    Step Two: Define the Problem 55
    Step Three: Study the Problem 61

Chapter 4. Determining What Happened and Why: The Search for Proximate Causes 77
    Step Four: Determine What Happened 77
    Step Five: Identify Contributing Process Factors 78
    Step Six: Identify Other Contributing Factors 79
    Step Seven: Measure—Collect and Assess Data on Proximate and Underlying Causes 82
    Step Eight: Design and Implement Interim Changes 85

Chapter 5. Identifying Root Causes 93
    Step Nine: Identify Which Systems Are Involved—The Root Causes 93
    Step Ten: Prune the List of Root Causes 99
    Step Eleven: Confirm Root Causes and Consider Their Interrelationships 99

Chapter 6. Designing and Implementing an Action Plan for Improvement 105
    Step Twelve: Explore and Identify Risk Reduction Strategies 105
    Step Thirteen: Formulate Improvement Actions 111
    Step Fourteen: Evaluate Proposed Improvement Actions 116
    Step Fifteen: Design Improvements 118
    Step Sixteen: Ensure Acceptability of the Action Plan 122
    Step Seventeen: Implement the Improvement Plan 122
    Step Eighteen: Develop Measures of Effectiveness and Ensure Their Success 128
    Step Nineteen: Evaluate Implementation of Improvement Efforts 130
    Step Twenty: Take Additional Action 130
    Step Twenty-one: Communicate the Results 131

Chapter 7. Tools and Techniques 147

Chapter 8. Root Cause Analysis Case Studies 175
    Using Aggregate Root Cause Analysis to Reduce Falls and Related Injuries 177
    Learning to Improve Safety: False-Positive Pathology Report Results in Wrongful Surgery 189

Glossary of Terms 199

Index 209

Introduction

Despite remarkable advances in almost every field of medicine, an age-old problem continues to challenge health care professionals—the occurrence of errors or *failures*—the term used increasingly instead of *errors*. When such failures harm individuals receiving health care services, the problem is extremely disturbing. Many, if not most, failures and sentinel events are the result of system and process problems. These problems inherently cause failures to occur and individuals to be harmed.

Such problems have been thrust into the limelight since the Institute of Medicine's (IOM's) watershed report, *To Err Is Human: Building a Safer Health System*. The report, which has been cited frequently in the media, states that 44,000 to 98,000 people die annually due to errors in inpatient hospital treatment. Total national costs (lost income, lost household production, disability, and health care costs) of preventable adverse events (medical errors resulting in injury) are estimated to be between $17 billion and $29 billion per year, of which health care costs represent more than one-half.[1]

The IOM report, however, was just the tip of the iceberg. Many other reports followed, illustrating the need to improve the quality of care being delivered in the United States. For example, researchers at Johns Hopkins Children's Center and the Agency for Healthcare Research and Quality reviewed 5.7 million records of patients under 19 years of age from 27 states who were hospitalized in 2000. Of the 52,000 children identified by the researchers as being harmed by unsafe medical care during their hospital stays, 4,483 suffered a fatal injury.[2] In addition, the researchers calculated that the additional medical cost of treating children injured by unsafe care exceeds $1 billion a year.

Although the reports shed light on the problem, it is virtually impossible to know how many patients suffer as a result of medical failures. The fact of the matter, however, is that any single failure, error, or sentinel event is a cause for concern. These events can result in tragedy for individuals served and their families, add cost to an already overburdened health care system, adversely affect the public's perception of an organization, and lead to litigation. They can also deeply affect health care professionals who are dedicated to helping individuals receiving care, treatment, or services. Why do these things happen?

The Current Health Care Environment

Health care continues to experience dramatic change. As health care organizations become more complex, their systems and processes are increasingly interdependent and are often interlocked and coupled. This increases the opportunity for failure and makes the recovery from failure by those involved more difficult. The rapid explosion of the medical knowledge base has made it increasingly challenging for practitioners to stay up-to-date. Despite technological advances and great gains in knowledge, health care systems are, and will continue to be, appropriately dependent on human intervention. The rigorous financial constraints imposed by managed care and the need to reduce health care expenditures have affected every type of health care organization. No organization is immune. Organization leaders are reassessing their work forces. Workloads are heavier, creating increased stress and fatigue for health care professionals. Caregivers are working in new settings and performing new functions, sometimes with minimal training. Skill mixes are shifting. In short, the health care environment is ripe for serious problems caused by systems failures.

Health care organizations are constantly evolving because of changes in reimbursement, new technology, regulatory requirements, and staffing levels. These modifications cause policies and procedures to change often and, in most cases, quickly. As a result, it is difficult to maintain consistency in processes and systems, which leads to variation. Often, this variation results in increased failure risk.

Instances of errors and sentinel events within health care organizations have been reported in the media with increasing regularity. These events cast a shadow on the public's trust of health care. People justifiably ask, "What's going on?" Failure detection, reduction, and prevention strategies are receiving needed new impetus as the health care industry recognizes the need for a proactive approach to reduce the risk of failure. Regulatory and accrediting agencies have responded to the public's concerns and the data outlining the medical errors by developing and revising standards and survey processes to emphasize that the primary focus is patient safety.

When an adverse outcome or sentinel event occurs, organizations must develop an understanding of the root causes of the event—the fundamental reasons a problem has occurred—and the interrelationship of causes. Next, the organization must implement improvement or redesign efforts to eliminate causative factors. It is clear that general knowledge about adverse events is limited, at best. General knowledge is even more limited in the area of proactive design or redesign of health care processes and systems. These aim to prevent, or at least minimize, the likelihood of future failures and to protect individuals from the harmful effects of failures when they do occur.

Purpose of the Book

Root Cause Analysis in Health Care: Tools and Techniques, Third Edition aims to help health care organizations prevent systems failures by using root cause analysis to identify causes of a sentinel event, to implement risk reduction strategies that decrease the likelihood of a recurrence of the event, and to identify effective and efficient ways of improving performance.

Root cause analysis is an effective technique most commonly used *after* an error has occurred to identify underlying causes. Failure mode and effects analysis (FMEA), also recommended by the Joint Commission, is a proactive technique used to prevent process and product problems *before* they occur. Health care organizations should learn both techniques to reduce the likelihood of adverse events. This book on root cause analysis and its companion on FMEA[3] outline both approaches in a step-by-step manner.

Root Cause Analysis in Health Care: Tools and Techniques, Third Edition provides readers with up-to-date information on the Joint Commission's Sentinel Event Policy and safety-related requirements. It also includes examples that guide the reader through application of root cause analysis to the investigation of specific types of sentinel events, such as medication errors, suicide, treatment delay, and elopement. For ease of access and use by root cause analysis teams, practical checklists and worksheets are offered at the end of each chapter.

This publication provides and explains the Joint Commission's framework for conducting a root cause analysis. It also helps organizations do the following:
- Identify the processes that could benefit from root cause analysis
- Conduct a thorough and credible root cause analysis
- Interpret analysis results
- Develop and implement an action plan for improvement
- Assess the effectiveness of risk reduction efforts
- Integrate root cause analysis with other programs

It is our hope that even without the occurrence of an adverse event, health care organizations will embrace the use of root cause analysis to investigate "near misses" in order to minimize the possibility of future failures and, thereby, to improve the care, treatment, and services provided at their facilities.

Overview of Contents

Root Cause Analysis in Health Care: Tools and Techniques, Third Edition provides health care organizations with practical, how-to information on conducting a root cause analysis. Twenty-one steps are described. Teams conducting a root cause analysis might not follow these steps in a sequential order. Often, numerous steps will occur simultaneously or the team will return to earlier steps before proceeding to the next step. It is critical for teams to customize or adapt the process to meet the unique needs of the team and organization. Appropriate tools for use in each stage of root cause analysis are identified in each chapter. A chapter-by-chapter look at the contents follows.

Chapter 1. Root Cause Analysis: An Overview provides an overview of root cause analysis. It describes variation, how proximate and root causes differ, when root cause analysis can be conducted, and the benefits of root cause analysis. One of the benefits involves effectively meeting Joint Commission requirements that relate to the management of sentinel events. The chapter also provides guidelines on the characteristics of a thorough and credible root cause analysis and action plan. It outlines the minimum scope of root cause analysis required by the Joint Commission for 10 specific types of sentinel events.

Chapter 2. Developing and Implementing a Policy and an Early Response Strategy for Sentinel Events describes the types of adverse events occurring in health care and the role that an organization's culture and leadership play in risk reduction and prevention. The Joint Commission's Sentinel Event Policy and requirements are provided in full, including a description of reportable and reviewable events. The chapter also includes practical guidelines on how an organization can develop its own sentinel event policy. It describes the need for root cause analysis and provides practical guidance on the early steps involved in responding to an adverse or sentinel event. These include prompt and appropriate care provided to the patient, risk containment to minimize the possibility of a similar event recurring immediately with other patients, event investigation so that the organization can explore exactly what occurred and learn from the event, and appropriate communication and disclosure to relevant parties.

Chapter 3. Preparing for Root Cause Analysis covers the early steps involved in performing a root cause analysis. The first of four hands-on workbook chapters, it describes how to organize a root cause analysis team, define the problem, and gather the information and measurement data to study the problem. Details are provided about team composition and meeting ground rules. The chapter also covers how to use information gleaned from the Joint Commission's Sentinel Event Database and accreditation requirements to identify problem areas in need of root cause analysis. Risk points and failure-prone systems are described, as is a method for developing an aim statement for a preliminary root cause analysis plan. Finally, the chapter provides guidance on recording information obtained during a root cause analysis, interviewing techniques, and gathering physical and documentary evidence.

Chapter 4. Determining What Happened and Why: The Search for Proximate Causes provides practical guidance on the next stage of root cause analysis—determining what happened and the reasons it happened. Organized in a workbook format, the chapter describes how to further define the event; identify process problems; determine which care processes are involved with the problem; and pinpoint the human, process, equipment, environmental, and other factors closest to the problem. The chapter also addresses how to collect and assess data on proximate and underlying causes. It provides guidance on choosing what to measure, describes indicators or measures, and guides teams through the process of ensuring that the data collected are appropriate to the desired measurement. In addition, the chapter describes the process of designing and implementing interim changes.

Chapter 5. Identifying Root Causes provides practical guidance, through workbook questions, on identifying or uncovering the root causes—the systems that lie underneath or behind sentinel events—and the interrelationship of the root causes to each other and other health care processes. Systems are explored and described, including human resources, information management, environment of care, leadership, communication, and uncontrollable factors. The chapter also addresses how to differentiate root causes and contributing causes. The most frequently occurring root causes identified by organizations that experienced a medication-related sentinel event, a restraint-related death, suicide in a 24-hour care setting, and wrong-site surgery are provided.

Chapter 6. Designing and Implementing an Action Plan for Improvement includes practical guidelines on how to design and implement an action plan—the improvement portion of a root cause analysis. During this stage, an organization identifies risk reduction strategies and designs and implements improvement strategies to address underlying systems problems. Characteristics of an acceptable action plan are provided, as is information on how to assess the effectiveness of improvement efforts. The chapter concludes with information on how to effectively communicate the results in improvement initiatives.

Chapter 7. Tools and Techniques presents the tools and techniques used during root cause analysis. Each tool profile addresses the purpose of the tool, the appropriate stage(s) of root cause analysis for the tool's use, simple steps for success, and tips for effective use. Tools and techniques include affinity diagrams, barrier analysis, brainstorming, cause-and-effect diagrams, change analysis, control charts, FMEA, fault tree analysis, flowcharts, Gantt charts, histograms, multivoting, Pareto charts, run charts, scatter diagrams, and timelines.

Chapter 8. Root Cause Analysis Case Studies presents root cause analyses that were originally published in the *Joint Commission Journal on Quality and Patient Safety*. The stories of real-life incidents at health care organizations are shared and the tools and techniques used to dig down to the root causes of the events are identified and explained.

Finally, the *Glossary* provides definitions of key terms used throughout the book.

A Word About Terminology

The terms *individual served, patient,* and *care recipient* all describe the individual, client, consumer, or resident who actually receives health care, treatment, and/or services. The term *care* includes care, treatment, services, rehabilitation, habilitation, or other programs instituted by an organization for individuals served.

Acknowledgments

Joint Commission Resources is deeply grateful to the many reviewers and content experts who have contributed their knowledge and expertise to this publication. This publication would not have been possible without the assistance of these individuals. JCR would also like to express its appreciation to writer John McCormack for the outstanding job he did revising this book.

References

1. Committee on the Quality of Health Care in America, Institute of Medicine: *To Err Is Human: Building a Safer Health System.* Washington, D.C.: National Academy Press, 2000.
2. Miller, Marlene R., and Chunliu Zhan: Pediatric Patient Safety in Hospitals: A National Picture in 2000. *Pediatrics* 113: 1741–1746, 2004.
3. Joint Commission Resources. *Failure Mode and Effects Analysis: Proactive Risk Reduction, Second Edition.* Oakbrook Terrace, IL: Joint Commission Resources, 2005.

Chapter 1
Root Cause Analysis: An Overview

What Is Root Cause Analysis?
Root cause analysis is a process for identifying the basic or causal factors that underlie variation in performance. Variation in performance can (and often does) produce unexpected and undesired adverse outcomes, including the occurrence or risk of a sentinel event. The Joint Commission defines *sentinel event* as an unexpected occurrence involving death or serious physical or psychological injury, or the risk thereof (*see* Chapter 2, page 25). A root cause analysis focuses primarily on systems and processes, not individual performance. To be successful, it must not assign blame. Rather, through the root cause analysis process, a team works to understand a process or processes, the causes or potential causes of variation, and process changes that make variation less likely to occur in the future.

A *root cause* is the most fundamental reason a failure, or a situation where performance does not meet expectations, has occurred. In common usage, the word *cause* suggests responsibility or a factor to blame for a problem. In this book, however, the use of the word *cause* implies no assignment of blame. Instead, the cause refers to a relationship or potential relationship between certain factors that enable a sentinel event to occur. Our focus in this publication is on a positive, preventive approach to system and process changes following a sentinel event or "near miss" sentinel event—one that almost occurred. Root cause analysis can do more than resolve that "A caused B." The process can also help an organization determine that "if we change A because we had a problem with it, we can reduce the possibility of B recurring or, in fact, prevent B from occurring in the first place."

When Can a Root Cause Analysis Be Performed?
Root cause analysis is most commonly used *reactively*—to probe the reason for a bad outcome or for failures that have already occurred. Root cause analysis can also be used to probe a "near miss"* event or as part of other performance improvement redesign initiatives, such as understanding variation in systematically collected data. The best root cause analyses look at the entire process and all support systems involved in a specific event to minimize overall risk associated with that process, as well as the recurrence of the event that prompted the root cause analysis.[1] The product of the root cause analysis is an *action plan* that identifies the strategies the organization intends to implement to reduce the risk of similar events occurring in the future.

Root cause analysis is also used increasingly by organizations as one step of a proactive risk reduction effort using failure mode and effects analysis (FMEA; *see* Chapter 7, pages 159-160). FMEA is a *proactive*, prospective approach used to prevent process and product problems before they occur. It provides a look not only at what problems could occur, but also at how severe the effects of those problems could be. Its goal is to prevent poor results, which in health care means *harm to patients*. One step of FMEA involves identifying the root causes of failures or *failure modes* created by special cause variation.[2] A root cause analysis approach is used at this point in the FMEA process.

---

* **Near miss** Used to describe any process variation that did not affect an outcome but for which a recurrence carries a significant change of a serious adverse outcome. Such a "near miss" falls within the scope of the definition of a sentinel event but outside the scope of those sentinel events that are subject to review by the Joint Commission under its Sentinel Event Policy.

This publication focuses on the use of root cause analysis to probe the underlying reasons for a sentinel event that has occurred or nearly occurred. In the nuclear power and aerospace industries, sentinel events are rare because they have been anticipated. Systems, often with significant redundancies, have been built to protect against them. In contrast, sentinel events in the health care environment, involving death or serious injury or the risk thereof, occur with relative frequency and tend to be handled largely in a reactive way.

Fundamentally, sentinel events in all environments provide two challenges:
1. To understand how and why the event occurred
2. To prevent the same or a similar event from occurring in the future through prospective process design or redesign

To meet these challenges, organizations must understand not only the *proximate causes* (the superficial, obvious, or immediate causes) of an event but more importantly the *underlying causes* (the causes that led to the proximate causes) and the interrelationship of causes. Root cause analysis helps organizations look underneath the apparent proximate causes to get at the root causes of a sentinel event (*see* Figure 1-1, page 9).

Conducting a root cause analysis has significant resource implications. A team approach, involving a full range of disciplines and departments in the process being studied, is mandatory, as described in Chapter 3. Organizations therefore will want to conduct root cause analysis principally to explore those events or possible events with a significant negative or potentially negative impact on care outcomes.

Variation and the Difference Between Proximate and Root Causes

Adverse or sentinel events involve unexpected variation in a process. When this variation occurs, there is a chance of a serious adverse outcome. As mentioned previously, root cause analysis is a process for identifying the basic or causal factors that underlie variation in performance. According to Webster's, *variation* is a change in the form, position, state, or qualities of a thing. Although a sentinel event is the result of an unexpected variation in a process, variation is inherent in every process. To reduce variation, it is necessary to determine its cause. In fact, variation can be classified by cause.

Common-cause variation, although inherent in every process, is a consequence of the way a process is designed to work. For example, an organization is examining the length of time required by the emergency department to obtain a routine radiology report. The time may vary depending on how busy the radiology service is or by when the report is requested. On a particular day, there may be many concurrent requests for reports, making it difficult for the radiology department to fill one specific request. Or, the report may have been requested between midnight and 6:00 A.M. when fewer radiology technologists are on duty. Variation in the process of providing radiology reports is inherent, resulting from common causes such as staffing levels and emergency department census. A process that varies only because of common causes is said to be stable. The level of performance of a stable process or the range of the common-cause variation in the process can be changed only by redesigning the process. Common-cause variation is systemic and endogenous, that is, produced from within. The organization needs to determine whether the amount of common-cause variation will be tolerated.

Another type of variation, *special-cause variation*, arises from unusual circumstances or events that may be difficult to anticipate and may result in marked variation and an unstable, intermittent, and unpredictable process. Special-cause variation is not inherently present in systems. It is exogenous, that is, produced from the outside, resulting from factors that are not part of the system as designed. Mechanical malfunction, intoxicated employees, floods, hurricanes, and other natural disasters are examples of special

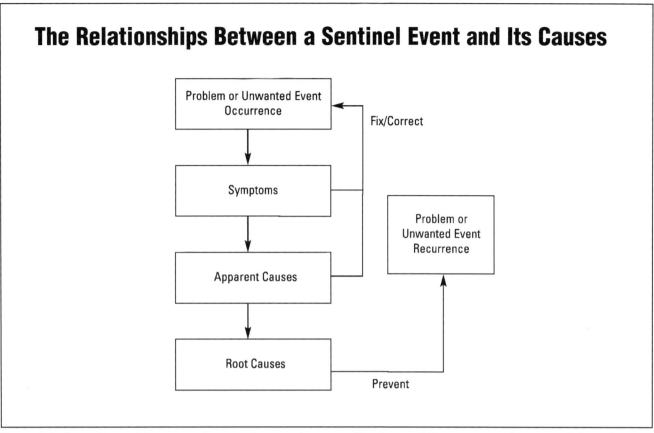

Figure 1-1. Correcting problems, symptoms, and apparent causes will not prevent the recurrence of an unwanted event. Only finding and resolving the root causes of the event can do this.
Source: Wilson P.F., Dell L.D., Anderson G.F.: *Root Cause Analysis: A Tool for Total Quality Management.* Milwaukee, WI: ASQC Quality Press, 1993, p 11. Used with permission.

causes that result in variation. Special causes should be identified and mitigated or eliminated, if possible. However, removing a special cause eliminates only that current abnormal performance in the process. It does not prevent the same special cause from recurring. For example, firing an intoxicated employee who failed to monitor a secluded patient or an overworked employee who was involved in a medication error does little to prevent the recurrence of the same error. Instead, organizations should investigate, understand, and address underlying common causes within their systems and processes such as personnel screening, staff education, staff supervision, information management, and communication.

Special causes in one process are usually the result of common causes in a larger system of which the process is a part. For example, mechanical breakdown of a piece of equipment used during surgery may indicate a problem with an organization's preventive maintenance activities. Similarly, an intoxicated employee and understaffed units indicate a problem with the organization's screening and hiring practices. Human resources practices must be examined for common-cause problems involving personnel screening and interview processes.

In health care, all the clinical and organizational processes and subprocesses associated with an event under review need to be delineated and evaluated to identify the degree of common-cause and/or special-cause variation. This process will assist organizations in identifying whether variation is due to clinical processes or organizational processes or both.

Any variation in performance, including a sentinel event, may be the result of a common cause, a special cause, or both. In the case of a sentinel event, the direct or proximate special cause could be uncontrollable factors. For example, a patient death results from a hospital's total loss of electrical power during a storm. This adverse outcome is clearly the result of a special cause in the operating room that is uncontrollable by the operating room staff. Staff members may be able to do little to prevent a future power outage and more deaths. However, the power outage and resulting death can also be viewed as the result of a common cause in the organization's system for preparing for and responding to a utility failure and other emergencies. Perhaps the backup generator that failed was located in the basement, which flooded during the storm, and the organization had no contingency plan for this adverse situation.

When looking at the chain of causation, proximate or direct causes tend to be nearest to the origin of the event. For example, proximate causes of a medication error may include a deteriorated drug, product mislabeling or misidentification, or an improper administration technique. By contrast, root causes are systemic and appear far from the origin of the event, often at the foundation of the processes involved in the event. For example, root causes of a medication error might include communication problems, inadequate staff training, or poor competence assessment.

Most root causes alone are not sufficient to cause a failure; rather, the combination of root causes sets the stage. For example, both failure to communicate changes in the conditions of a patient and failure to perform adequate assessments can be root causes of a patient's fall from bed. Organizations that are successful in effectively identifying all the root causes and their interactions can eliminate a plethora of risks when redesigning processes.[3] Elimination of one root cause reduces the likelihood of that one very specific adverse outcome occurring again. However, if the organization misses the five other root causes, it is possible that they could interact to cause a different, but equally adverse, outcome. Chapter 5 describes how organizations can identify and explore the interrelationship of multiple root causes.

Benefits of Root Cause Analysis

Why conduct root cause analysis? All health care organizations experience problems of varying persistence and magnitude. Organizations can improve their operations and the care they provide through probing and addressing the roots of such problems. Individual accountability for faulty performance should not be the focus. Rather, the focus should be on systems—how to improve systems to prevent the occurrence of sentinel events or problems. This approach involves digging into the organization's systems to find new ways to do things. It is focused on answering the question, "What should we *do* to prevent this in the future?" not "What should we *have done* to prevent this from having occurred?" The emphasis is on improving systems.

Thus, root cause analysis helps organizations identify risk or weak points in processes, underlying or systemic causes, and corrective actions. Moreover, information from root cause analyses shared between and among organizations can help to prevent future sentinel events. Knowledge shared in the health care field can contribute to proactive improvement efforts and results.

In addition, organizations use root cause analysis to meet Joint Commission requirements relating to the management of sentinel events. Each Joint Commission accreditation manual contains sentinel event requirements in a separate chapter called "Sentinel Events" at the beginning of the accreditation manuals and also in the "Improving Organization Performance" and "Leadership" chapters. The requirements as they generally appear are shown in Sidebar 1-1, pages 11-12. Requirements relevant to safety, performance improvement, and health care error reduction appear in Sidebar 1-2, page 13.

Sidebar 1-1. Joint Commission Sentinel Event Requirements

Improving Organization Performance Requirements: Performance improvement (PI) involves measuring the functioning of important processes and services, and, when indicated, identifying changes that enhance performance. An important aspect of improving organization performance is effectively reducing factors that contribute to unanticipated adverse events and/or outcomes that can be caused by poorly designed systems, system failures, or errors.

Identifying, reporting, analyzing, and managing sentinel events can help the organization prevent sentinel events. Leaders define and implement such a program as part of the process to measure, assess, and improve the organization's performance. **PI.2.30**, which states that processes for identifying and managing sentinel events are defined and implemented, lists those processes as the following:

- Defining "sentinel event" and communicating this definition throughout the organization. (At a minimum, the organization's definition includes those events subject to review under the Joint Commission's Sentinel Event Policy as published in current accreditation manuals and may include any process variation which does not affect the outcome or result in an adverse event, but for which a recurrence carries significant chance of a serious adverse outcome or results in an adverse event, often referred to as a "near miss.") **(PI.2.30, EP 1)**
- Reporting sentinel events through established channels in the organization and, as appropriate, to external agencies in accordance with law and regulation **(PI.2.30, EP 2)**
- Conducting thorough and credible root cause analyses that focus on process and system factors **(PI.2.30, EP 3)**
- Creating, documenting, and implementing a risk-reduction strategy and action plan that includes measuring the effectiveness of process and system improvements to reduce risk **(PI.2.30, EP 4)**
- Implementing the processes **(PI.2.30, EP 5)**

Data help determine performance improvement priorities. As stated in **PI.1.10**, the data collected for high priority and required areas are used to monitor the stability of existing processes, identify opportunities for improvement, identify changes that lead to improvement, or sustain improvement. Data collection helps identify specific areas that require further study. These areas are determined by considering the information provided by the data about process stability, risks, sentinel events, and priorities set by leaders.

PI.2.20 states that undesirable patterns or trends in performance are analyzed, and an analysis is performed to make changes that improve performance and patient safety and reduce the risk of sentinel events for the following:

- All confirmed transfusion reactions, if applicable to the organization **(PI.2.20, EP 4)**
- All serious adverse drug events, if applicable and as defined by the organization **(PI.2.20, EP 5)**
- All significant medication errors, if applicable and as defined by the organization **(PI.2.20, EP 6)**
- All major discrepancies between preoperative and postoperative (including pathologic) diagnoses **(PI.2.20, EP 7)**
- Adverse events or patterns of adverse events during moderate or deep sedation and anesthesia use **(PI.2.20, EP 8)**
- Hazardous conditions **(PI.2.20, EP 9)**
- Staffing effectiveness issues **(PI.2.20, EP 10)**

Sidebar 1-1. Joint Commission Sentinel Event Requirements, *continued*

Leadership Requirements: The Joint Commission's accreditation requirements recognize that leadership is a vital element in planning, directing, coordinating, providing, and improving care, treatment, and services to respond to the needs of individuals and improve health care outcomes as well as to create a framework for organizations to respond to sentinel events. **LD.4.40** states that leaders must ensure that the patient safety program at their organization includes the following regarding sentinel events:

- Definition of the scope of the program's oversight, typically ranging from no-harm, frequently occurring "slips" to sentinel events with serious adverse outcomes **(LD.4.40, EP 2)**

- Procedures for immediately responding to system or process failures, including care, treatment, or services for the affected individual(s), containing risk to others, and preserving factual information for subsequent analysis **(LD.4.40, EP 4)**

- Clear systems for internal and external reporting of information about system or process failures **(LD.4.40, EP 5)**

- Defined responses to various types of unanticipated adverse events and processes for conducting proactive risk assessment/risk reduction activities **(LD.4.40, EP 6)**

- Defined support systems* for staff members who have been involved in a sentinel event **(LD.4.40, EP7)**

- Reports, at least annually, to the health care organization's governance or authority on system or process failures and actions taken to improve safety, both proactively and in response to actual occurrences **(LD.4.40, EP 8)**

In addition, as stated in **LD.4.20**, leaders must ensure that new or modified services or processes are designed well. The design of new or modified services or processes should incorporate the following:

- The needs and expectations of patients, staff, and others **(LD.4.20, EP 1)**

- The results of performance improvement activities, when available **(LD.4.20, EP 2)**

- Information about potential risks to patients, when available **(LD.4.20, EP 3)**

- Current knowledge, when available and relevant (for example, practice guidelines, successful practices, information from relevant literature and clinical standards) **(LD.4.20, EP 4)**

- Information about sentinel events, when available and relevant **(LD.4.20, EP 5)**

- Testing and analysis to determine whether the proposed design or redesign is an improvement **(LD.4.20, EP 6)**

- Leadership collaboration with staff and appropriate stakeholders to design services **(LD.4.20, EP 7)**

---

* Support systems provide individuals with additional help and support as well as additional resources through the human resources function or an employee assistance program. Support systems recognize that conscientious health care workers who are involved in sentinel events are themselves victims of the event and require support. Support systems also focus on the process rather than blaming the involved individuals.

Sidebar 1-2. Requirements Relevant to Safety, Performance Improvement, and Health Care Error Reduction

- The integrity of decisions is based on identified care, treatment, and service needs of the patients. **(RI.1.30)**

- Information from data analysis is used to make changes that improve performance and patient safety and reduce the risk of sentinel events. **(PI.3.10)**

- An ongoing, proactive program for identifying and reducing unanticipated adverse events and safety risks to patients is defined and implemented. **(PI.3.20)**

- Communication is effective throughout the organization. **(LD.3.60)**

- The leaders set expectations, plan, and manage processes to measure, assess, and improve the organization's governance, management, clinical, and support activities. **(LD.4.10)**

- The leaders set performance improvement priorities and identify how the health care organization adjusts priorities in response to unusual or urgent events. **(LD.4.50)**

- The leaders allocate adequate resources for measuring, assessing, and improving the health care organization's performance and improving patient safety. **(LD.4.60)**

  ○ Sufficient staff is assigned to conduct activities for performance improvement and safety improvement. **(LD.4.60, EP 1)**

  ○ Adequate time is provided for staff to participate in activities for performance improvement and safety improvement. **(LD.4.60, EP 2)**

  ○ Adequate systems are provided to support activities for performance improvement and safety improvement. **(LD.4.60, EP 3)**

  ○ Staff is trained in performance improvement and safety improvement approaches and methods. **(LD.4.60, EP 4)**

- The leaders measure and assess the effectiveness of the performance improvement and safety improvement activities. **(LD.4.70)**

  ○ The leaders assess the adequacy of the human, information, physical, and financial resources allocated to support performance improvement and safety improvement activities. **(LD4.70, EP 3)**

The leadership requirements related to sentinel events detail how an organization's patient safety program should address sentinel events, including the following: defining "sentinel event" and communicating this definition throughout the organization, reporting sentinel events through established channels and to external agencies in accordance with law and regulation, conducting root cause analyses, and using a risk-reduction strategy and action plan. In addition, the leadership requirements address how new or modified services or processes should be designed and systematically monitored, analyzed, and improved to enhance health care outcomes of individuals.

The sentinel event performance improvement requirements address what an organization should do when it experiences a sentinel event to ensure patient safety and comply with law and regulations. The requirement gives the organization flexibility to define what would be considered a sentinel event within the organization. At a minimum, an organization's definition must include those events that are subject to review under the Sentinel Event Policy. The reporting requirements of any relevant agency should be considered by the organization in formulating its definition. Leaders must set the stage by establishing a culture conducive to performance improvement and must be involved in the process of identifying and managing sentinel events through root cause analysis. A plan must also be established to address improvement opportunities and identify who is responsible for implementing and assessing the plan. In addition, these requirements state that data should be collected for high priority and required areas to monitor the stability of existing processes, identify opportunities for improvement, identify changes that lead to improvement, or sustain improvement. Finally, these requirements state that undesirable patterns or trends in performance should be analyzed and an analysis should be performed to make changes that improve performance and patient safety and reduce the risk of sentinel events.

Through these requirements, accredited organizations are expected to identify and respond appropriately to all sentinel events occurring in the organization or associated with services that the organization provides or provides for. An appropriate response includes conducting a thorough and credible root cause analysis, implementing improvements to reduce risk, and monitoring the effectiveness of those improvements.

The Root Cause Analysis and Action Plan: Doing It Right

How can a health care organization ensure that its root cause analysis and action plan provide an appropriate response to a sentinel event occurring in the organization, as outlined in the requirements? A root cause analysis is considered acceptable if it has the following characteristics:

- The analysis focuses primarily on systems and processes, not individual performance.
- The analysis progresses from special causes in clinical processes to common causes in organizational processes.
- The analysis repeatedly digs deeper by asking "Why?"; then, when answered, asks "Why?" again, and so on.
- The analysis identifies changes that could be made in systems and processes (either through redesign or development of new systems or processes) that would reduce the risk of such events occurring in the future.
- The analysis is thorough and credible.

To be thorough, the root cause analysis must include the following:

- A determination of the human and other factors most directly associated with the sentinel event and the process(es) and systems related to its occurrence
- An analysis of the underlying systems and processes through a series of "Why?" questions to determine where redesign might reduce risk
- An inquiry into all areas appropriate to the specific type of event
- An identification of risk points and their potential contributions to this type of event
- A determination of potential improvement in processes or systems that would tend to decrease the likelihood of such events in the future, or a determination, after analysis, that no such improvement opportunities exist

To be credible, the root cause analysis must do the following:
- Include participation by the leadership of the organization and by individuals most closely involved in the processes and systems under review
- Be internally consistent (that is, not contradict itself or leave obvious questions unanswered)
- Provide an explanation for all findings of "not applicable" or "no problem"
- Include consideration of any relevant literature

The product of a root cause analysis is an *action plan* that identifies the strategies the organization intends to implement to reduce the risk of similar events occurring in the future. The plan should address responsibility for implementation, oversight, pilot testing (as appropriate), timelines, and strategies for measuring the effectiveness of the actions.

An action plan will be considered acceptable if it does the following:
- Identifies changes that can be implemented to reduce risk or formulates a rationale for not undertaking such changes
- Identifies, in situations where improvement actions are planned, who is responsible for implementation, when the action will be implemented (including any pilot testing), and how the effectiveness of the actions will be evaluated

All root cause analyses and action plans are considered and treated as confidential by the Joint Commission.

Data gathered by the Joint Commission between January 1995 and December 2004 from review of more than 2,900 sentinel events indicate that about 90% of these events fall into the following categories: patient suicide; op/post-op complication; wrong-site surgery; medication error; delay in treatment; patient death/injury in restraints; patient fall; assault/rape/homicide; transfusion error; perinatal death/loss of function; patient elopement; fire; ventilator death/injury; anesthesia-related event; infection-related event; medical equipment-related event; maternal death; abduction of any individual receiving care, treatment, or services; discharge of an infant to the wrong family; and utility systems-related event. Review of the root cause analyses of these events has allowed the Joint Commission to identify patterns for risk reduction activities.

Figure 1-2, page 16, shows the minimum scope of root cause analysis for 10 specific types of sentinel events. An organization experiencing a sentinel event in one of these categories is expected to conduct a thorough and credible root cause analysis, which, at a minimum, inquires into each of the areas identified for that category of event. This inquiry should determine that there is, or is not, opportunity with the associated system(s), process(es), or function(s) to redesign or otherwise take action to reduce risk. A root cause analysis submitted in response to a sentinel event in one of the listed categories is considered unacceptable if it does not, at a minimum, address each of the areas specified for that type of event.

Due to the potential impact on the accreditation process, an organization should seek clarification of any questions about the Joint Commission's Sentinel Event Policy and the requirements for a root cause analysis by calling the Joint Commission's Sentinel Event Hotline (*see* Sidebar 1-3, page 17). Organizations may also wish to use the Joint Commission's Web site at http://www.jcaho.org, which includes detailed information on the Sentinel Event Policy and root cause analysis (*see* Sidebar 1-4, page 18).

Table 1-1, page 17, outlines the high-level key tasks involved in performing a thorough and credible root cause analysis and action plan. Overall, a thorough and credible root cause analysis should do the following:
- Be clear (understandable information)
- Be accurate (validated information and data)
- Be precise (objective information and data)
- Be relevant (focus on issues related or potentially related to the sentinel event)

Minimum Scope of Root Cause Analysis for Specific Types of Sentinel Events

Root Cause Analysis Matrix

	Suicide (24° care)	Med. Error	Proced. Cmplic.	Wrong site surg.	Treatment delay	Restraint death	Elopement death	Assault/ rape/ hom.	Transfusion death	Infant abduction
Behavioral assessment process[1]	X					X	X	X		
Physical assessment process[2]	X		X	X	X	X	X			
Patient identification process		X		X					X	
Patient observation procedures	X					X	X	X	X	
Care planning process	X		X			X	X			
Continuum of care	X				X	X				
Staffing levels	X	X	X	X	X	X	X	X	X	X
Orientation & training of staff	X	X	X	X	X	X	X	X	X	X
Competency assessment / credentialing	X	X	X		X	X	X	X	X	X
Supervision of staff		X	X		X	X			X	
Communication with patient/family	X			X	X	X	X			X
Communication among staff members	X	X	X	X	X	X			X	X
Availability of information	X	X	X	X	X	X			X	
Adequacy of technological support		X	X							
Equipment maintenance/ management		X	X			X				
Physical Environment[4]	X	X	X				X	X	X	X
Security systems and processes	X						X	X		X
Control of medications: storage/access		X							X	
Labeling of medication		X							X	

1. Includes the process for assessing patient's risk to self (and to others, in cases of assault, rape, or homicide where a patient is the assailant).
2. Includes search for contraband.
3. Includes supervision of physicians-in-training.
4. Includes furnishings; hardware (e.g., bars, hooks, rods); lighting; distractions.

Figure 1-2. The Joint Commission requires detailed inquiry into these areas when conducting a root cause analysis for the specified type of sentinel event. Inquiry into areas not checked (or not listed) should be conducted as appropriate for the specific event under review.

Table 1-1. Conducting a Root Cause Analysis and Implementing an Action Plan

- Assign an interdisciplinary team to assess the sentinel event.
- Establish a way to communicate progress to senior leadership.
- Create a high-level work plan with target dates, responsibilities, and measurement strategies.
- Define all the issues clearly.
- Brainstorm all possible or potential contributing causes and their interrelationships.
- Sort and analyze the cause list.
- For each cause, determine which process(es) and system(s) it is a part of and the interrelationship of causes.
- Determine whether the causes are special causes, common causes, or both.
- Begin designing and implementing changes while finishing the root cause analysis.
- Assess the progress periodically.
- Repeat activities as needed (for example, brainstorming).
- Be thorough and credible.
- Focus improvements on the larger system(s).
- Redesign to eliminate the root cause(s) and the interrelationship of root causes that can create an adverse outcome.
- Measure and assess the new design.

Sidebar 1-3. Sentinel Event Hotline

The Joint Commission established the Sentinel Event Hotline to respond to inquiries about the Sentinel Event Policy. For more information about the hotline, visit http://www.jcaho.org/accredited+organizations/hospitals/sentinel+events/index.htm. The Sentinel Event Hotline phone number is 630/792-3700. The hotline is staffed from 8:30 A.M. to 5:00 P.M. Central Standard Time, Monday through Friday.

Callers can speak with a member of the Joint Commission staff about the Sentinel Event Policy and about whether an event meets the criteria to be considered a sentinel event under the policy.

- Be complete (cover all causes and potential causes)
- Be systematic (methodically conducted)
- Possess depth (ask and answer all of the relevant "Why" questions)
- Possess breadth of scope (cover all possible systemic factors wherever they occur)

The Joint Commission's framework for a root cause analysis and action plan appears as Figure 1-3, pages 20-23. This framework, to be used extensively in Chapters 4 through 6, provides a solid foundation for root cause analyses and action plans. The tool selection matrix, found in Chapter 7 as Figure 7-1 (page 148), can also be used as a guide to ensure that an organization considers and selects the most appropriate tools and techniques for root cause analysis.

Sidebar 1-4. Sentinel Event Information on the Web

The Joint Commission's Web site includes detailed information geared toward helping health care organizations comply with the Joint Commission's Sentinel Event Policy. To access sentinel event–related information from the Joint Commission's home page (http://www.jcaho.org), click "Sentinel Events" found under "Top Spots." This links to the "Sentinel Event Resource Index," which includes the following searchable topics:

- **Sentinel Event Policy and Procedures:** A description of the Joint Commission's Sentinel Event Policy and procedures, including self-reporting and root cause analysis

- **Sentinel Event Statistics:** Current statistical information on sentinel events by type, setting, source, outcome, total self-reported, total non–self-reported, and methods for review of organizations' responses to sentinel events

- **Facts about the Sentinel Event Policy:** Important information about the Sentinel Event Policy covering topics such as self-reporting of sentinel events and confidentiality of information

- *Sentinel Event Alert*: Newsletter about sentinel events, their causes, and error and reduction strategies

- **Sentinel Event Advisory Group:** Group of experienced physicians, nurses, pharmacists, and other patient safety experts appointed by the Joint Commission in April 2002 to advise the Joint Commission in the development of its first set of National Patient Safety Goals (NPSGs). The Sentinel Event Advisory Group does the following:
    - Annually recommends core and program-specific NPSGs and related specific implementation requirements for adoption by the Joint Commission Board of Commissioners
    - Reviews draft patient safety recommendations for potential publication in the Joint Commission's periodic *Sentinel Event Alert* advisory and advises Joint Commission staff as to the evidence for and face validity of these recommendations, as well as their practicality and cost of implementation
    - Advises Joint Commission staff as to the acceptability of alternative practices implemented by or being considered by accredited organizations in lieu of implementing the specific requirements associated with the Joint Commission's individual NPSGs.
    - Recommends topics for future consideration in *Sentinel Event Alert*

- **Sentinel Event Forms and Tools**
    - Affirmation Statement
    - Framework for Conducting a Root Cause Analysis
    - Tool to Assist Organizations in the Completion of the Framework for Conducting a Root Cause Analysis
    - Process Flow Chart (for event reporting and responses)
    - Root Cause Analysis Matrix
    - Self-Report Form

- **Voluntarily Reportable Sentinel Events:** Examples of sentinel events that are voluntarily reportable to the Joint Commission as well as events that are not reportable

- **Sentinel Event Reporting Alternatives:** Information about Alternatives 1, 2, 3, and 4 for sharing sentinel event–related information with the Joint Commission

- **Glossary of Sentinel Event Terms:** Terms and definitions related to sentinel events

References

1. Croteau R.J., Schyve P.M.: Chapter 7: Proactively error-proofing health care processes. In: Spath P (Ed): *Error Reduction in Health Care*. San Francisco, CA: Jossey-Bass Publishers, 2000, pp. 179–198.
2. Joint Commission Resources. *Failure Mode and Effects Analysis: Proactive Risk Reduction, Second Edition.* Oakbrook Terrace, IL: Joint Commission Resources, 2005.
3. Root cause analysis: Identifying multiple root causes is key to improving performance. *Joint Commission Perspectives on Patient Safety*™ 2(2):4–5, Feb. 2002.

Root Cause Analysis in Health Care: Tools and Techniques, Third Edition

A Framework for a Root Cause Analysis and Action Plan in Response to a Sentinel Event

Page 1 of 4

Level of Analysis		Questions	Findings	Root Cause?	Ask "Why?"	Take Action
What happened?	Sentinel Event	What are the details of the event? (Brief description)		▓	▓	▓
		When did the event occur? (Date, day of week, time)		▓	▓	▓
		What area/service was impacted?				
Why did it happen?	The process or activity in which the event occurred.	What are the steps in the process, as designed? (A flow diagram may be helpful here)				
What were the most proximate factors?	Human factors	What steps were involved in (contributed to) the event?				
(Typically "special cause" variation)		What human factors were relevant to the outcome?				
	Equipment factors	How did the equipment performance affect the outcome?				
	Controllable environmental factors	What factors directly affected the outcome?				
	Uncontrollable external factors	Are they truly beyond the organization's control?		▓	▓	
	Other	Are there any other factors that have directly influenced this outcome?				
		What other areas or services are impacted?				

Figure 1-3. This framework outlines several questions that may be used to probe for systems problems underlying problematic processes. In each area, consider whether and how the factors can be improved, as well as the pros and cons of expending resources to make improvements.

A Framework for a Root Cause Analysis and Action Plan in Response to a Sentinel Event, *continued*

Page 2 of 4

This template is provided as an aid in organizing the steps in a root cause analysis. Not all possibilities and questions will apply in every case, and there may be others that will emerge in the course of the analysis. However, all possibilities and questions should be fully considered in your quest for "root cause" and risk reduction.

As an aid to avoiding "loose ends," the three columns on the right are provided to be checked off for later reference:

- Root Cause? should be answered "yes" or "no" for each finding. A root cause is typically a finding related to a process or system that has a potential for redesign to reduce risk. If a particular finding that is relevant to the event is not a root cause, be sure that it is addressed later in the analysis with a "Why?" question. Each finding that is identified as a root cause should be considered for an action and addressed in the action plan.
- Ask "Why?" should be checked off whenever it is reasonable to ask why the particular finding occurred (or didn't occur when it should have) – in other words, to drill down further. Each item checked in this column should be addressed later in the analysis with a "Why?" question. It is expected that any significant findings that are not identified as root causes themselves have "roots."
- Take action? Should be checked for any finding that can reasonably be considered for a risk reduction strategy. Each item checked in this column should be addressed later in the action plan. It will be helpful to write the number of the associated Action Item on page 3 in the Take Action? column for each of the findings that requires an action.

Level of Analysis		Questions	Findings	Root Cause?	Ask "Why?"	Take Action
Why did that happen? What systems and processes underlie those proximate factors? (Common cause variation here may lead to special cause variation in dependent processes)	Human Resources issues	To what degree are staff properly qualified and currently competent for their responsibilities?				
		How did actual staffing compare with ideal levels?				
		What are the plans for dealing with contingencies that would tend to reduce effective staffing levels?				
		To what degree is staff performance in the operant process(es) addressed?				

A Framework for a Root Cause Analysis and Action Plan in Response to a Sentinel Event, *continued*

Page 3 of 4

Level of Analysis	Questions	Findings	Root Cause?	Ask "Why?"	Take Action
Information management issues	How can orientation and in-service training be improved?				
	To what degree is all necessary information available when needed? Accurate? Complete? Unambiguous?				
	To what degree is communication among participants adequate?				
Environmental management issues	To what degree was the physical environment appropriate for the processes being carried out?				
	What systems are in place to identify environmental risks?				
	What emergency and failure-mode responses have been planned and tested?				
Leadership issues: - Corporate culture	To what degree is the culture conducive to risk identification and reduction?				
- Encouragement of communication	What are the barriers to communication of potential risk factors?				
- Clear communication of priorities	To what degree is the prevention of adverse outcomes communicated as a high priority? How?				
Uncontrollable factors	What can be done to protect against the effects of these uncontrollable factors?				

A Framework for a Root Cause Analysis and Action Plan in Response to a Sentinel Event, *continued*

Page 4 of 4

Action Plan	Risk Reduction Strategies	Measures of Effectiveness
For each of the findings identified in the analysis as needing an action, indicate the planned action expected, implementation date, and associated measure of effectiveness. OR. …	Action Item #1:	
If after consideration of such a finding, a decision is made not to implement an associated risk reduction strategy, indicate the rationale for not taking action at this time.	Action Item #2:	
Check to be sure that the selected measure will provide data that will permit assessment of the effectiveness of the action.	Action Item #3:	
	Action Item #4:	
Consider whether pilot testing of a planned improvement should be conducted.	Action Item #5:	
Improvements to reduce risk should ultimately be implemented in all areas where applicable, not just where the event occurred. Identify where the improvements will be implemented.	Action Item #6:	
	Action Item #7:	
	Action Item #8:	

Cite any books or journal articles that were considered in developing this analysis and action plan:

Chapter 2
Developing and Implementing a Policy and an Early Response Strategy for Sentinel Events

Root cause analysis plays a key role in the identification and prevention of sentinel events. What is a sentinel event and how does it differ from other events, incidents, or occurrences that take place routinely in health care organizations? What role does organization culture play in the identification and prevention of adverse events? What does the Joint Commission require when a sentinel event occurs? What types of events are reviewable by the Joint Commission and what types are nonreviewable? What types of events require root cause analysis? What issues should be considered as an organization develops its own sentinel event policy? What should an organization do following a sentinel event? Who must be notified? What are the legal and ethical considerations of disclosure to patients? The answer to some of these questions really is, "It depends." Although there are few hard-and-fast rules, some general guidelines can be useful. This chapter provides such guidelines while urging readers to consult additional sources of information as needed.

Sentinel Events and the Range of Adverse Events in Health Care

The Joint Commission defines *sentinel event* as an unexpected occurrence resulting in death or serious physical or psychological injury, or the risk thereof. Serious injury specifically includes loss of limb or function. The phrase *or the risk thereof* includes any process variation for which a recurrence would carry a significant chance of a serious adverse outcome for a recipient of care, treatment, or services. Such events are called sentinel because they signal the need for immediate investigation and response. According to Webster's, the word *sentinel* means "one who watches or guards." An event is sentinel because it involves an unexpected variation in a process or an outcome and demands notice. Organizations must watch their care processes and guard against such an event.

Sentinel events commonly result from errors of commission or omission. An error of *commission* occurs as a result of an action taken, for example, when an improper technique is used to restrain a patient and the patient asphyxiates or when surgery is performed on the wrong limb. Other examples include a medication given by the incorrect route, an infant discharged to the wrong family, or electro-convulsive therapy administered to the wrong patient.

An error of *omission* occurs when an action is *not* taken, for example, when a delayed diagnosis results in a patient's death, when a medication dose ordered is not given, when a physical therapy treatment is missed, or when a patient suicide is associated with a lapse in carrying out frequent observation. Errors of omission and commission may or may not lead to adverse outcomes. For example, a patient in seclusion is not monitored during the first two hours. The staff corrects the situation by beginning regular observations as specified in organization policy. The possibility of failure is present, however, and the mere fact that the staff does not follow organization policy regarding seclusion, and thereby violates acceptable professional standards, signals the occurrence of a failure requiring study to ensure that it does not happen again. In this case, the error of omission was insufficient monitoring. If the patient suffers serious physical or psychological harm during seclusion, the sentinel event is his or her adverse outcome. By definition, sentinel events require further investigation each time they occur.

Fortunately, the majority of failures (whether called events, incidents, or occurrences) cause no harm. For example, missed medication dosages or dosages administered at the wrong time rarely result in death or serious harm. Similarly, a missed observation of a patient in seclusion rarely results in the patient's death or serious harm. However, the presence of these events may signal the presence of a much larger problem. Organizations should integrate information about such events as part of their ongoing data collection and analysis.

Sometimes failures result in no serious harm but are significant enough to be considered a "near miss." For example, a drug dosage is administered to a patient via the incorrect route, such as intravenously rather than orally. The patient feels the effect but survives and suffers no permanent harm. However, the patient could have suffered harm and perhaps would even be expected to with a similar error. It is good practice for organizations to conduct a root cause analysis or some other form of intensive analysis for such important single events, but such events usually are not reportable under the Joint Commission's Sentinel Event Policy described later in the chapter (*see* pages 27-38). The process used by the organization to review sentinel events should be reviewed by the organization as it completes its Periodic Performance Review (PPR) and during the organization's normal triennial survey (or, from 2006 on, during its unannounced full accreditation survey).

Sentinel events—that is, important single events that should trigger intense investigation—are a subset of all adverse events. Of those sentinel events, an even smaller subset at the tip of the pyramid are the sentinel events that are reviewable under the Joint Commission's Sentinel Event Policy. These include failures involving patient deaths and permanent loss of function. Figure 2-1, page 27, shows the relationship of reviewable sentinel events to both sentinel events in general and broader categories of adverse events. Table 2-1, page 31, lists examples of sentinel events reviewable by the Joint Commission. See page 30 for a complete description of reviewable sentinel events. As described in Chapter 1, organizations are required to conduct a thorough and credible root cause analysis and action plan for each of these sentinel events. The Joint Commission reviews the analysis and plan and adds the information to its database, to be described in more detail later. Table 2-2, page 32, provides a list of nonreviewable events.

Leadership, Culture, and Sentinel Events

For the sentinel event policy to be effective, the culture of an organization and the role of its leaders need to support the prevention and identification of sentinel events.

Leaders must be deeply committed to patient safety and to ensuring that members of their organization truly embody their missions, visions, and values. They play a critical role in fostering an organization culture in which sentinel event reporting, root cause analyses, and proactive risk reduction are encouraged. Reporting helps an organization to start the process of both identifying root causes and developing and implementing risk reduction strategies. Understanding that continuous improvement is essential to an organization's success, leaders must have the authority and willingness to allocate resources for root cause analyses and improvement initiatives. They must ensure that the processes for identifying and managing sentinel events are defined and implemented (*see* the corresponding performance improvement requirement in Sidebar 1-1, pages 11-12). They must be willing and able to set an example for the organization and empower staff to identify and bring about necessary change. Effective leaders empower staff *throughout* the organization to acquire and apply the knowledge and skills needed to continuously improve processes and services.

An organization's response to a sentinel event speaks volumes about the culture of that organization. Its response can also significantly influence the likelihood of similar events occurring in the future. Historically,

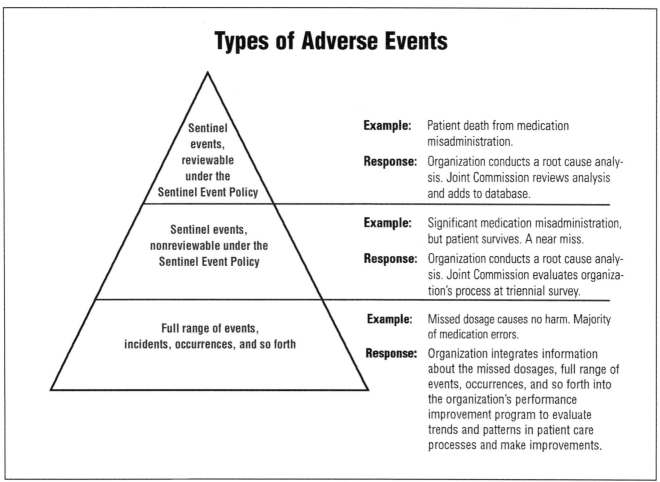

Figure 2-1. This triangular figure shows the relationship of Joint Commission–reviewable sentinel events to both sentinel events in general and the broader category of adverse events.

the response to sentinel events has been to identify the individual(s) most closely associated with the event and take some form of punitive action. "Who did it?" has, too often, been the first question asked, rather than "Why did it happen?"

The organization that routinely asks "Why?" rather than "Who?" will, over time, learn more about the quality and safety of the care it is providing—as well as its sentinel events, "near misses," and hazardous conditions—and will better understand the relationship between its staff and the processes, systems, and environment in which they function.[1]

Through commitment to performance improvement, patient safety, and proactive risk reduction, leaders build an organization culture that values change, creativity, teamwork, and communication. Teams provide much of the impetus for performance improvement. Communication and information flow throughout the organization to foster a barrier-free learning environment.

The Joint Commission's Sentinel Event Policy

When developing and implementing a sentinel event policy of their own, organizations must understand the Joint Commission's Sentinel Event Policy. A description follows here. Figure 2-2, page 28, provides a graphic representation of the sentinel event process flow. The information provided here is current as of the date of publication. Changes to the policy are published in *Joint Commission Perspectives*® and on the

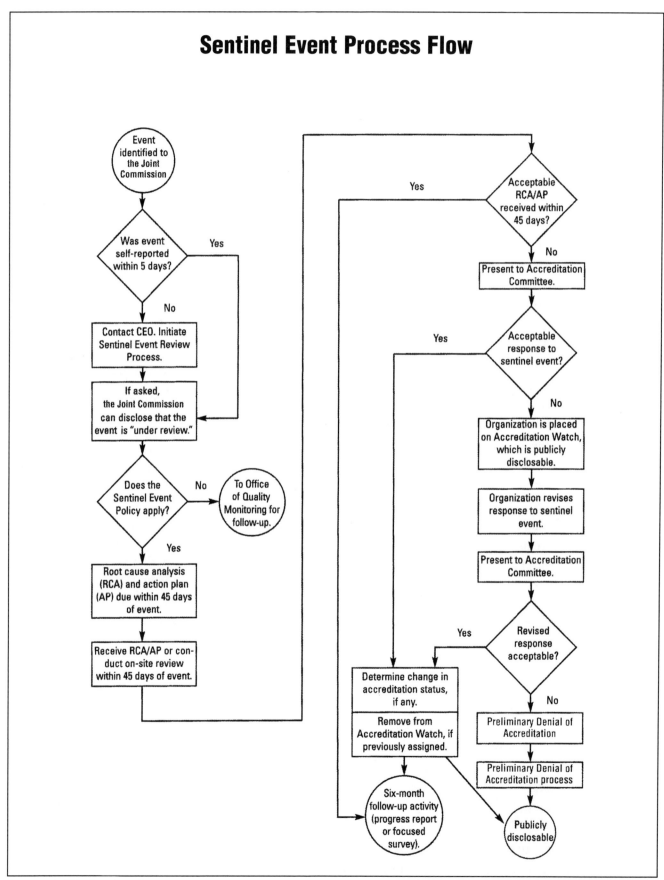

Figure 2-2. This flowchart displays the steps in the implementation of the Joint Commission's Sentinel Event Policy and its procedures.

Perspectives home page of the Joint Commission Resources Web site at http://www.jcrinc.com/perspectives.

In support of its mission to improve the quality of health care provided to the public, the Joint Commission includes the reviews of organizations' activities in response to sentinel events in its accreditation process, including all full accreditation surveys and random unannounced surveys.

The four goals of the policy are to do the following:
1. Have a positive impact in improving patient care, treatment, and services and preventing sentinel events
2. Focus the attention of an organization that has experienced a sentinel event on understanding the causes that underlie that event and on changing the organization's systems and processes to reduce the probability of such an event in the future
3. Increase the general knowledge about sentinel events, their causes, and strategies for prevention
4. Maintain the confidence of the public and accredited organizations in the accreditation process

Survey Process

In conducting an accreditation survey, Joint Commission surveyors seek to evaluate the organization's compliance with the applicable requirements discussed in Chapter 1 and to score those requirements based on performance throughout the organization over time (for example, the preceding 12 months for a full accreditation survey). Under the sentinel event requirements, accredited organizations are expected to identify and respond appropriately to *all* sentinel events (as defined by the organization) occurring in the organization or associated with services that the organization provides, or provides for. An appropriate response includes conducting a timely, thorough, and credible root cause analysis; implementing improvements to reduce risk; and monitoring the effectiveness of those improvements.

Surveyors are instructed not to seek out specific sentinel events beyond those already known to the Joint Commission. The intent is to evaluate compliance with the relevant leadership and performance improvement requirements—that is, how the organization responds to sentinel events when they occur. However, if a surveyor becomes aware of a sentinel event while on site, the organization is required to provide follow-up information that indicates that a root cause analysis and action plan have been conducted. If in the course of conducting an on-site survey a surveyor identifies a potentially reviewable sentinel event that has not previously been reported to the Joint Commission, he or she will take the following steps:

- Inform the CEO that the event has been identified
- Inform the CEO the event will be reported to the Joint Commission for further review and follow-up under the provisions of the Sentinel Event Policy

During the on-site survey, the surveyor(s) will assess the organization's compliance with sentinel event–related standards in the following ways:

- Review the organization's process for responding to a sentinel event
- Interview the organization's leaders and staff about their expectations and responsibilities for identifying, reporting, and responding to sentinel events
- Ask for and review an example of a root cause analysis that has been conducted in the past year to assess the adequacy of the organization's process for responding to a sentinel event. Additional examples may be reviewed if needed to more fully assess the organization's understanding of, and ability to conduct, root cause analyses. In selecting an example, the organization may choose a "closed case" or a "near miss" to demonstrate its process for responding to a sentinel event.

Surveyors also review the effectiveness and sustainability of organization improvements in systems and processes in response to sentinel events previously evaluated under the Joint Commission's Sentinel Event Policy.

Reviewable Sentinel Events

The subset of sentinel events that falls within the scope of the Joint Commission's Sentinel Event Policy and is subject to review by the Joint Commission includes any occurrence that meets any of the following criteria:

- The event has resulted in an unanticipated death or major permanent loss of function, not related to the natural course of the patient's illness or underlying condition[*,†]
- The event is one of the following (even if the outcome was not death or major permanent loss of function not related to the natural course of the patient's illness or underlying condition):
  - Suicide of any individual receiving care, treatment, or services in a staffed around-the-clock setting or within 72 hours of discharge
  - Unanticipated death of a full-term infant
  - Abduction of any individual receiving care, treatment, or services
  - Discharge of an infant to the wrong family
  - Rape[‡]
  - Hemolytic transfusion reaction involving administration of blood or blood products having major blood group incompatibilities
  - Surgery on the wrong patient or wrong body part[§]

The Joint Commission Web site (http://www.jcaho.org) has the most up-to-date information about options currently available for organizations that have experienced a sentinel event.

Again, Table 2-1, page 31, lists examples of reviewable sentinel events.

How the Joint Commission Becomes Aware of a Sentinel Event

Each health care organization is encouraged, but not required, to report to the Joint Commission any sentinel event meeting the preceding criteria for reviewable sentinel events. Alternatively, the Joint Commission may become aware of a sentinel event by some other means, such as communication from a patient, family member, or employee of the organization or through the media.

If the Joint Commission becomes aware (either through voluntary self-reporting or otherwise) of a sentinel event meeting the preceding criteria that has occurred in an accredited organization, the organization is expected to do the following:

- Prepare a thorough and credible root cause analysis and action plan within 45 calendar days of the event or of becoming aware of the event

---

[*] *Major permanent loss of function* means sensory, motor, physiologic, or intellectual impairment not present on admission requiring continued treatment or lifestyle change. When major permanent loss of function cannot be immediately determined, applicability of the policy is not established until either the patient is discharged with continued major loss of function or two weeks have elapsed with persistent major loss of function, whichever occurs first.

[†] A distinction is made between an adverse outcome that is primarily related to the natural course of a patient's illness or underlying condition (not reviewed under the Sentinel Event Policy) and a death or major permanent loss of function that is associated with the treatment (including "recognized complications") or lack of treatment of that condition, or otherwise not clearly and primarily related to the natural course of the patient's illness or underlying condition (reviewable). In indeterminate cases, the event is presumed reviewable and the organization's response is reviewed under the Sentinel Event Policy according to the prescribed procedures and time frames without delay for additional information such as autopsy results.

[‡] *Rape*, as a reviewable sentinel event, is defined as unconsented sexual contact involving a patient and another patient, staff member, or other perpetrator while being treated or on the premises of the health care organization, including oral, vaginal, or anal penetration or fondling of the patient's sex organ(s) by another individual's hand, sex organ, or object. One or more of the following must be present to determine reviewability:
- Any staff-witnessed sexual contact as described previously
- Sufficient clinical evidence obtained by the organization to support allegations of unconsented sexual contact
- Admission by the involved perpetrator that sexual contact, as described previously, occurred on the premises

[§] All events of surgery on the wrong patient or wrong body part are reviewable under the policy, regardless of the magnitude of the procedure or the outcome.

> ## Table 2-1. Examples of Joint Commission–Reviewable Sentinel Events
>
> - Any patient death, paralysis, coma, or other major permanent loss of function associated with a medication error
> - Any suicide of a patient in a setting where the patient is housed around-the-clock, including suicides following elopement from such a setting
> - Any elopement, that is unauthorized departure, of a patient from an around-the-clock care setting resulting in a temporally related death (suicide or homicide) or major permanent loss of function
> - Any procedure on the wrong patient, wrong side of the body, or wrong organ
> - Any intrapartum (related to the birth process) maternal death
> - Any perinatal death unrelated to a congenital condition in an infant having a birth weight greater than 2,500 grams
>
> - Assault, homicide, or other crime resulting in patient death or major permanent loss of function
> - A patient fall that results in death or major permanent loss of function as a direct result of the injuries sustained in the fall
> - Hemolytic transfusion reaction involving major blood group incompatibilities
>
> Note: An adverse outcome that is *directly* related to the natural course of a patient's illness or underlying condition, for example, terminal illness present at the time of presentation, is **not** reportable **except** for suicide in, or following elopement from, a 24-hour care setting.
>
> This list may not apply to all settings.

- Submit to the Joint Commission its root cause analysis and action plan, or otherwise provide for Joint Commission evaluation of its response to the sentinel event under an approved protocol, within 45 calendar days of the known occurrence of the event

The Joint Commission then determines whether the root cause analysis and action plan are acceptable. If the root cause analysis or action plan is not acceptable, the organization is at risk for being placed on Accreditation Watch by the Accreditation Committee (*see* page 34). Joint Commission staff are available to discuss the thoroughness and credibility of the root cause analysis with organizations.

An organization that experiences a sentinel event that does *not* meet the criteria for review under the Sentinel Event Policy is still expected to complete a root cause analysis. However, the root cause analysis need *not* be made available to the Joint Commission.

Reasons for Reporting a Sentinel Event to the Joint Commission

Although self-reporting of a sentinel event is not required, there are several advantages for organizations that report a sentinel event, including the following:

- Reporting the event enables the addition of the lessons learned from the event and root cause analysis to be added to the Joint Commission's Sentinel Event Database, thereby contributing to the general knowledge about sentinel events and reducing risk for such events in many other organizations.
- Early reporting provides an opportunity for discussion with Joint Commission staff during the development of the root cause analysis and action plan.

> ### Table 2-2. Examples of Sentinel Events *Not* Reviewable by the Joint Commission
>
> - Any "near miss"
> - Full return of limb or bodily function to the same level as prior to the adverse event by discharge or within two weeks of the initial loss of said function
> - Any sentinel event that has not affected a recipient of care (patient, client, resident)
> - Medication errors that do not result in death or major permanent loss of function
> - Suicide other than in an around-the-clock care setting or following elopement from such a setting
> - A death or loss of function following a discharge "against medical advice" (AMA)
> - Unsuccessful suicide attempts
> - Unintentionally retained foreign body without major permanent loss of function
> - Minor degrees of hemolysis with no clinical sequelae
>
> Note: In the context of its performance improvement activities, an organization may choose to conduct intensive assessment, for example, root cause analysis, for some nonreporting events.

- The organization's message to the public that it is doing everything possible to ensure that such an event will not happen again is strengthened by its acknowledged collaboration with the Joint Commission to understand how the event happened and what can be done to reduce the risk of such an event in the future.

There is no difference in the expected response, time frames, or review procedures, whether the organization voluntarily reports the event or the Joint Commission becomes aware of the event by some other means.

Voluntary Reporting of Sentinel Events to the Joint Commission

If an organization wishes to report an occurrence in the subset of sentinel events that are subject to review by the Joint Commission, the organization is asked to complete a sentinel event reporting form (*see* Figure 2-3, page 33). This form can be accessed online at http://www.jcaho.org/accredited+organizations/hospitals/sentinel+events/forms+and+tools/index.htm. In addition to obtaining copies of the sentinel event reporting form online, organizations can obtain copies of the form by calling the Sentinel Event Hotline at 630/792-3700 or the Office of Quality Monitoring at 630/792-5642.

The organization sends this form to the Joint Commission's Office of Quality Monitoring by mail or by facsimile (630/792-5636). The Office of Quality Monitoring can also be accessed online at http://www.jcaho.org/general+public/public+input/report+a+complaint/off_qm.htm. Each organization is contacted within five days to finalize root cause analysis due date, receive a case number, and share the method chosen to review the root cause analysis.

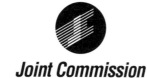

Joint Commission
on Accreditation of Healthcare Organizations

Accredited Organization Self-Reported Sentinel Event

_____ _____
Full Name of Accredited Organization   Organization ID Number (HCO#)

_____
Street Address   City   State   Zip Code

_____
Date of Incident

Summary of Incident: (Please describe the event but do not include names of patient(s), caregiver(s), or other individual(s) involved in the event.)

_____
_____
_____
_____
_____
_____

Select method of sharing sentinel event–related information:

_____ Mailing Root Cause Analysis

_____ Alternative #1   _____ Alternative #2

_____ Alternative #3   _____ Alternative #4

_____
Sentinel Event Contact (please print full name)   Phone #   E-mail address

_____
Title

_____
Signature   Date   Fax #

Figure 2-3. A Joint Commission–accredited organization that experiences a reportable sentinel event can complete this reporting form to apprise the Joint Commission of the event and the status of the root cause analysis.

Reviewable Sentinel Events That Are Not Reported by the Organization

If the Joint Commission becomes aware of a sentinel event subject to review under the Sentinel Event Policy that was not reported to the Joint Commission by the organization, the chief executive officer of the organization is contacted, and a preliminary assessment of the sentinel event is made. For occurrences meeting the criteria for review under the Sentinel Event Policy, the organization is required to submit or make available an acceptable root cause analysis and action plan, or choose an approved protocol, within 45 calendar days of the event or becoming aware of the event.

Initial On-Site Review of a Sentinel Event

An initial on-site review of a sentinel event is usually not conducted unless it is determined that there is a potential ongoing threat to patient health or safety or potentially significant noncompliance with major Joint Commission requirements. If an on-site (for-cause) review is conducted, the organization is billed an appropriate amount to cover the costs of conducting such a survey.

Disclosable Information

If, during the 45-day analysis period, the Joint Commission receives an inquiry about the accreditation status of an organization that has experienced a *reviewable* sentinel event, the organization's accreditation status is reported in the usual manner without making reference to the sentinel event. If the inquirer specifically references the sentinel event, the Joint Commission acknowledges that it is aware of the event and is working with the organization through the sentinel event review process. If the Joint Commission receives an inquiry about a specific sentinel event at an organization after the 45-day analysis period has passed, the Joint Commission either acknowledges that the organization met the requirements for responding to the sentinel event or states that the organization has been placed on Accreditation Watch if the organization has not met the requirements for responding to the sentinel event.

Finally, if an inquiry is made when the organization has not fully complied with the requirements for responding to a sentinel event but has not yet been placed on Accreditation Watch, the organization's accreditation status is reported in the usual manner without making reference to the sentinel event.

Accreditation Watch Designation

Accreditation Watch is an attribute of an organization's Joint Commission accreditation status. It publicly acknowledges the collaborative efforts by the organization and the Joint Commission to understand the factors underlying a sentinel event and to implement appropriate changes to reduce the risk of such events in the future.

A health care organization is placed on Accreditation Watch when a reviewable sentinel event has occurred and has come to the Joint Commission's attention, and when a thorough and credible root cause analysis of the sentinel event and action plan have not been completed within a specified time frame. Although Accreditation Watch status is not an official accreditation category, it can be publicly disclosed by the Joint Commission.

Required Response to a Reviewable Sentinel Event

If the Joint Commission becomes aware of a sentinel event in an accredited organization, and the occurrence meets the criteria for review under the Sentinel Event Policy, the organization is required to submit or otherwise make available an acceptable root cause analysis and action plan—or otherwise provide for Joint Commission evaluation of its response to the sentinel event using an approved protocol—within 45 calendar days of the event or of becoming aware of the event. If the determination has been made that an event is reviewable under the Sentinel Event Policy, and more than 45 days have elapsed since the known occurrence of the event, the organization is allowed 15 days for its response.

If the organization fails to submit or otherwise make available an acceptable root cause analysis and action plan—or otherwise provide for Joint Commission evaluation of its response to the sentinel event under an approved protocol—within the 45 calendar days (or within 15 calendar days, if the 45 days have already elapsed), the organization is at risk for being placed on Accreditation Watch if the sentinel event subsequently becomes known to the Joint Commission.

Initiation of Accreditation Watch
If the Joint Commission becomes aware that an organization has experienced a reviewable sentinel event, but the organization fails to submit or otherwise make available an acceptable root cause analysis and action plan—or otherwise provide for Joint Commission evaluation of its response to the sentinel event under an approved protocol—within 45 days of the event or of becoming aware of the event, a recommendation is made to the Accreditation Committee to place the organization on Accreditation Watch. If the Joint Commission's Accreditation Committee places the organization on Accreditation Watch, the organization is then permitted an additional 15 days to submit an acceptable root cause analysis and action plan or otherwise provide for Joint Commission evaluation of its response to the sentinel event under an approved protocol.

The organization will be offered assistance in performing a root cause analysis of the event. In all cases of organization refusal to permit review of information regarding a reviewable sentinel event in accordance with the Sentinel Event Policy and its approved protocols, the initial response by the Joint Commission is assignment of Accreditation Watch. Continued refusal may result in loss of accreditation.

Submission of Root Cause Analysis and Action Plan
An organization that experiences a sentinel event subject to review under the Sentinel Event Policy is asked to submit two documents: (a) the completed root cause analysis, which includes enough detail to demonstrate that the analysis is thorough and credible, and (b) the resulting action plan that describes the organization's risk reduction strategies and plan for evaluating their effectiveness. A framework for a root cause analysis and action plan (*see* Figure 1-3, pages 20-23) is available to organizations as an aid in organizing the steps in a root cause analysis and developing an action plan. It is also available on the Joint Commission's Web site at http://www.jcaho.org.

The root cause analysis and action plan are *not* to include the patient's name or the names of caregivers involved in the sentinel event.

Reporting Options
If an organization has concerns about increased risk of legal exposure as a result of sending the root cause analysis documents to the Joint Commission, the following alternative approaches to the Joint Commission review of the organization's response to the sentinel event are acceptable:

1. Review of root cause analysis and action plan documents brought to Joint Commission headquarters by organization staff and then taken back to the organization on the same day. The organization is assessed a charge sufficient to cover the cost of staff time and room use.

2. An on-site visit by a specially trained surveyor to review the root cause analysis and action plan. The organization is assessed a charge sufficient to cover the average direct costs of the visit.

3. An on-site visit by a specially trained surveyor to review the root cause analysis and findings, without directly viewing the root cause analysis documents, through a series of interviews and review of relevant documentation. For purposes of this review activity, "relevant documentation" includes, at a minimum, any documentation relevant to the organization's process for responding to sentinel events and the action plan resulting from the analysis of the subject sentinel event. The latter serves as the basis for appropriate follow-up activity. The organization is assessed a charge sufficient to cover the average direct costs of the visit.

4. Where the organization affirms that it meets specified criteria respecting the risk of waiving legal protection for root cause analysis information shared with the Joint Commission, an on-site visit is made by a specially trained surveyor to conduct interviews and review relevant documentation to obtain information about the following:

- The process the organization uses in responding to sentinel events

- The relevant policies and procedures preceding and following the organization's review of the specific event, and the implementation thereof, sufficient to permit inferences about the adequacy of the organization's response to the sentinel event. In addition, the surveyor conducts a standards-based survey of the patient care and organization management functions relevant to the sentinel event under review. The organization is assessed a charge sufficient to cover the average direct costs of the visit.

A request for review of an organization's response to a sentinel event using any of these alternative approaches must be received by the Joint Commission within at least five days of the self-report of a reviewable event or of the initial communication by the Joint Commission to the organization that it has become aware of a reviewable sentinel event.

The Joint Commission's Response

Staff assesses the acceptability of an organization's response to a reviewable sentinel event, including the thoroughness and credibility of any root cause analysis information reviewed and the organization's action plan. If the root cause analysis and action plan are found to be thorough and credible, the response is accepted and an appropriate follow-up activity is assigned. A written report on progress related to the action plan is required by the six-month point.

If the response is unacceptable, staff provides consultation to the organization on the criteria that have not yet been met and allows an additional 15 calendar days beyond the original 45-day submission period for the organization to resubmit its response. This additional time is provided only if the organization's initial submission of its root cause analysis and action plan was within the 45-day time frame.

If the response continues to be unacceptable, staff recommends to the Accreditation Committee that the organization be placed on Accreditation Watch and be required to address the inadequacies and submit, or make available for review, a new root cause analysis and action plan, or otherwise provide for further Joint Commission evaluation of its response to the event within 15 days of notification that the Accreditation Committee has found the response to be unacceptable and has placed the organization on Accreditation Watch.

Depending on the nature and extent of the inadequacies of the organization's initial response to the sentinel event, the Joint Commission determines whether an on-site visit should be made to assist the organization in conducting an appropriate root cause analysis and developing an action plan.

If, on review, the organization's response is still not acceptable, or the organization fails to respond, staff recommends to the Accreditation Committee that the organization be placed in Preliminary Denial of Accreditation. If approved by the Accreditation Committee, this accreditation status is considered publicly disclosable information and the process for resolution of Preliminary Denial of Accreditation is initiated.

When the organization's response, initial or revised, is found to be acceptable, the Joint Commission issues an *Official Accreditation Decision Report* that does the following:

- Reflects the Accreditation Committee's determination to continue or modify the organization's current accreditation status and terminate the Accreditation Watch if previously assigned

- Assigns an appropriate follow-up activity, typically a measure of success or follow-up visit to be conducted within six months

Follow-Up Activity

The follow-up activity assesses, based on applicable standards, an organization's response to additional relevant information obtained since completion of the root cause analysis, the implementation of system and process improvements identified in the action plan, the means by which the organization continues to assess the effectiveness of those efforts, the organization's response to data collected to measure the effectiveness of the actions, and the resolution of any outstanding requirements for improvement. The follow-up activity is conducted when the organization believes it can demonstrate effective implementation—but no later than six months following receipt of the *Official Accreditation Decision Report*.

A decision to maintain or change the organization's accreditation status as a result of the follow-up activity or to assign additional follow-up requirements is based on existing decision rules unless otherwise determined by the Accreditation Committee.

Each sentinel event evaluated under the Joint Commission's Sentinel Event Policy is reviewed at the organization's next full accreditation survey. This review focuses on the implementation of risk reduction strategies and the effectiveness of these actions.

The Sentinel Event Database

To achieve the third goal of the Sentinel Event Policy—to increase the general knowledge about sentinel events, their causes, and strategies for prevention—the Joint Commission collects and analyzes data from the review of sentinel events, root cause analyses, action plans, and follow-up activities. These data and information form the content of the Joint Commission's Sentinel Event Database.

In response to concerns about potential increased legal exposure for accredited organizations through the sharing of such information with the Joint Commission, the Joint Commission has committed to the development and maintenance of this Sentinel Event Database in a fashion that excludes organization, caregiver, and patient identifiers. Three major categories of data elements are included in the Joint Commission's cumulative database:

- Sentinel event data (without organization, caregiver, or patient identifiers)
- Root cause data
- Risk reduction data

Aggregate data relating to root causes and risk reduction strategies for sentinel events that occur with significant frequency form the basis for future error-prevention advice to health care organizations through *Sentinel Event Alert* and other media.

Handling Sentinel Event-Related Documents

Upon completing the review of any submitted root cause analysis and action plan, and then abstracting the required data elements for the Joint Commission's Sentinel Event Database, the original root cause analysis documents and any copies are destroyed, or, upon request, the original documents are returned to the organization. Handling these sensitive documents is restricted to specially trained staff in accordance with procedures designed to protect the confidentiality of the documents.

The action plan resulting from the analysis of the sentinel event is initially retained to serve as the basis for the follow-up activity. After the action plan has been implemented to the satisfaction of the Joint Commission, as determined through follow-up activities, the Joint Commission destroys the action plan.

Legal Concerns over Confidentiality

The basic tenets of the Sentinel Event Policy* are that an organization must perform a root cause analysis in response to a sentinel event and that if the Joint Commission becomes aware of the event, the

---

* The Joint Commission's General Counsel is available to answer questions about the Sentinel Event Policy. Find the General Counsel's contact information online at http://www.jcaho.org/contact+us/directory.htm.

organization must share relevant root cause analysis information with the Joint Commission. Almost all organizations experiencing sentinel events appear to be moving quickly to address the first tenet. However, serious concerns regarding the potential discoverability of sentinel event–related information shared with the Joint Commission have created a significant barrier in meeting the second tenet for organizations in many states.

In response to these concerns, the Joint Commission, after being advised by an outside group of health care lawyers from various groups, including some state hospital association lawyers, has identified four alternative ways for a health care organization to report, and the Joint Commission to review, information regarding the organization's response to a sentinel event. These alternatives, outlined on page 35, are intended to reduce the exposure of sensitive sentinel event–related information while preserving an environment that encourages the candid and thorough assessment of the root causes of sentinel events. The Joint Commission believes that the confidentiality needs of accredited organizations can be well met by one or more of these alternatives; however, there are no absolute guarantees that these alternatives *ensure* the confidentiality of privileged sentinel event–related information shared with the Joint Commission.*

The Joint Commission firmly believes that the sharing of information between the Joint Commission and accredited organizations should not waive confidentiality protection granted to any particular information by any particular state law. If requested, the Joint Commission would strongly make this point in any court or legislature. As of the publication of this book, the Joint Commission knows of no such waiver case.

Again, with the advice of outside lawyers, the Joint Commission has also identified contractual agreements that may substantively address the legal concerns regarding the potential waiver of confidentiality protections in certain states. These agreements involve having the health care organization do the following:

- Identify the Joint Commission as a participating entity in the organization's peer review or quality improvement activities

  or

- Appoint the Joint Commission to the organization's peer review or quality improvement committee

These agreements suggest that the Joint Commission should not be viewed as an external third party in the limited context of an intensive assessment of a sentinel event and, therefore, no waiver of confidentiality protections should occur by sharing sentinel event–related information with the Joint Commission. These agreements may permit an organization to readily comply with the Sentinel Event Policy (that is, submit its root cause analysis and action plan to the Joint Commission) or otherwise serve to enhance the protections afforded by the alternatives.

The Joint Commission is actively pursuing federal and state legislation to enhance protections for the confidentiality of sentinel event–related information shared with national accrediting bodies. Questions regarding legal protections of sentinel event information can be directed to the Department of Legal Affairs. Contact information for the Department of Legal Affairs can be found online at http://www.jcaho.org/contact+us/directory.htm.

Developing a Sentinel Event Policy

The first step in developing an organization's sentinel event policy† is to determine which events warrant root cause analysis. The Joint Commission expects accredited organizations to identify and respond

---

* The fourth alternative does not involve the Joint Commission reviewing or being told about the privileged root cause analysis.

† Please note that although the Joint Commission requires organizations to define "sentinel event" and communicate its definition throughout the organization, the Joint Commission does not require organizations to develop a sentinel event policy. The information provided here is intended to provide advice on how an organization might develop a sentinel event policy if it wishes to do so.

appropriately to all sentinel events, as defined by the Joint Commission, occurring in the organization or associated with services that the organization provides, or provides for. This helps to ensure improvement of the organization's processes. As outlined earlier, appropriate response includes a thorough and credible root cause analysis, implementation of improvements to reduce risk, and monitoring of the effectiveness of those improvements.

Performance improvement standard PI.2.30 (outlined in Chapter 1, page 11) requires each accredited organization to define *sentinel event* for its own purposes in establishing mechanisms to identify, report, and manage these events. While this definition must be consistent with the Joint Commission's general definition of a sentinel event, as provided on page 25, accredited organizations have some latitude in setting more specific parameters to define *unexpected, serious,* and *the risk thereof*.

For example, an organization may wish to define a sentinel event as a serious event involving staff and visitors as well as patients. Or an organization may wish to include the following:
- All unusual events, even though they may result in only minor adverse outcomes
- All events that must be reported to an external agency
- Events with potential for an adverse public, economic, or regulatory impact

An organization's definition should include those events that are subject to review under the Sentinel Event Policy (*see* page 30). The definition should also apply organizationwide and should appear in writing in an organization plan or policy. Through a collaborative process, organization leaders as well as medical, nursing, and administrative staff should develop the definitions or categories of events that warrant root cause analysis.

In developing the organization's sentinel event policy, leaders may also address the process for reporting a sentinel event to leadership, how "near misses" are to be handled, and the process for the ongoing management of sentinel events and prevention efforts. Leaders may also wish to identify the following:
- The individual responsible for receiving initial notification of a sentinel event
- The individual responsible for assessing whether or not the event warrants an in-depth root cause analysis based on the organization's definition of a sentinel event (this may be the same individual, for example, a physician, risk manager, quality assurance coordinator, or program manager)
- How this individual communicates the need for in-depth investigation and necessary information to a team of individuals responsible for performing the root cause analysis
- The individual responsible for facilitating and overseeing a team-based root cause analysis process

Leaders should also address confidentiality, discoverability, and disclosure. Information obtained during the investigation of sentinel events through root cause analysis or other techniques is often highly sensitive. The organization's sentinel event policy should address how confidentiality will be protected. The policy should also address the procedure for obtaining legal consultation to protect relevant documents such as meeting minutes, reports, and conversations from discovery in the event of a future lawsuit. The policy should be clear on whether the state in which the organization operates protects the details of a sentinel event investigation from discovery under the organization's quality management, peer review, or risk management programs.

Following the development of the organization's sentinel event policy, leaders should ensure that all staff and physicians are knowledgeable about the organization's sentinel event policies and procedures. In-service programs and new staff and physician orientation should address the organization's sentinel event policy on a regular and continuing basis. This includes regular updates concerning sentinel events published by the

Joint Commission and additional issues that may be identified through the organization's compliance with the National Patient Safety Goals. Table 2-3, page 41, outlines the steps described in this section.

Early Response Strategies

An organization has just experienced a sentinel event leading to a serious adverse outcome. What must be done? Following the occurrence of a sentinel event, staff members must simultaneously take a number of actions. An organization's sentinel event policy should outline early response strategies. These include the following:

- Providing prompt and appropriate care for the affected patient(s)
- Containing the risk of an immediate recurrence of the event
- Preserving the evidence

Appropriate Care

The prompt and proper care of a patient who has been affected by a sentinel event should be the providers' and staff members' first concern following the event. Care could involve, as appropriate, stabilizing the patient, arranging for his or her transportation to a health care facility for surgery or testing, providing medications, taking actions to prevent further harm, and reversing the harm that has occurred, if possible. When appropriate, physicians should obtain medical consultation related to the adverse event and arrange to receive necessary follow-up information.

Communication with the family (discussed further on page 46) is vital during the time period immediately following the event.

Risk Containment

Following a sentinel event, the organization must respond by immediately containing the risk of the event occurring again. If a patient suffered a stroke as a result of the misadministration of a drug, are other patients at risk for similar injuries? If so, the organization must take immediate action to safeguard patients from a repetition of the unwanted occurrence. Risk management texts, articles appearing in the literature, and associations such as the American Society for Healthcare Risk Management* can provide detailed guidance.

Preservation of Evidence

To learn from a failure and understand why it occurred, it is critical to know exactly what occurred. Preserving the evidence is essential to this process. Immediate steps should be taken to secure any biological specimens, medications, equipment, medical or other records, and any other material that might be relevant to investigating the failure.[2] In medication-related events, syringes of recently used medications and bottles of medications should be preserved and sequestered. Because such evidence may be discarded as a part of routine operations, such as when empty vials are thrown into trash cans, it is critical to obtain and preserve it promptly. Protocols established by the health care organization should specify the steps to be taken to preserve relevant evidence following a sentinel event.

Event Investigation

Documentation and appropriate communication and disclosure to relevant parties must also be considered immediately following the occurrence of a sentinel event.

Documentation

Proper medical record documentation of errors or sentinel events is critical for the continuity of care. Documentation tips appear in Table 2-4, page 42. A thoroughly completed incident-reporting form can be very helpful during the early stages of event investigation and during Steps 2 through 4 of root cause analysis (Chapters 3 and 4). Health care organizations use a variety of occurrence or incident-reporting tools and generally have a policy and procedure covering their use. Forms or questionnaires may be general in nature, covering all types of adverse

---

* The American Society for Healthcare Risk Management can be found online at http://www.ashrm.org or by phone at 312/422-3980.

Table 2-3. Steps in Developing a Sentinel Event Policy

- Define *sentinel event*, setting specific parameters for what constitutes *unexpected, serious*, and *the risk thereof*. Remember that the general definition must be consistent with the Joint Commission's definition.
- Include the definition of sentinel event in writing in an organization plan or policy.
- Determine which events warrant root cause analysis using a collaborative process.
- Determine the process for reporting a sentinel event to leadership.
- Determine the process for reporting the event to external agencies.
- Determine how near misses are to be handled.
- Determine how the ongoing management of sentinel events and prevention efforts are to be handled.
- Address how confidentiality of information related to sentinel events will be protected.
- Address the procedure for obtaining legal consultation to protect relevant documents.
- Educate all staff and physicians about the policy and procedures; ensure ongoing education.
- Review the policy annually and revise information, such as reviewable sentinel events, the process for reporting sentinel events, confidentiality issues, legal issues, and relevant staff education, as appropriate.

events, or be specific to event types. Figure 2-4, page 43, is a sample medication error occurrence report.

Communication and Disclosure

With the occurrence of a sentinel event, personnel involved in the incident should promptly notify those responsible for error reporting and investigation within the organization. Supervisors, quality and risk management professionals, and administrators should be informed. These individuals can determine how best to notify other parties, including the press and external agencies such as federal, state, and local authorities. Legal counsel should be sought early in the process. Counsel can provide guidance in how to discuss the situation with the family, how to prevent disclosure of potentially defamatory information, and how to handle media relations.[3]

One recommendation states that organizations maintain two lists of key people to contact following a sentinel event: key individuals *within* the organization and individuals *outside* the organization.[4] Both lists should be kept up-to-date with current telephone numbers and should be accessible to managers, supervisors, and members of a crisis management team. A sample sentinel event notification checklist appears as Figure 2-5, page 44.

Responding to media queries through organization protocols helps to avert complications related to patient confidentiality, legal discovery, and heat-of-the-moment coverage.[5] Notification requirements should be reflected in organization policies and procedures. These should include policies for communication with the patient and family, described in the following paragraphs.

> ### Table 2-4. Tips for Documenting Adverse Events
>
> - Assign the most involved and knowledgeable member(s) of the health care team to record factual statements of the event in the patient's record.
>
> - Record any medical follow-up completed, planned, or needed.
>
> - Avoid writing information in the medical record that is unrelated to the care of the patient (such as "legal office notified").
>
> - Avoid writing derisive comments about other providers; in the event of a disagreement with another clinician, the health care team should document only the basis for their treatment recommendations.
>
> - When adding information to the patient's record after an adverse event has occurred, mark the entry with the actual date it is written; do not "backdate" any entries.
>
> - Beware of creating entries that appear self-serving—especially explanations intended solely to justify someone's actions.

Source: Keyes C.: Responding to adverse events. *Forum* 18(1):3, 1997. Used with permission.

A provider's communication and disclosure with relevant parties following the occurrence of an event that led or could have led to patient injury is critical. Relevant parties include the following:

- Patients and families affected by the event
- Colleagues who could provide clarification, support, and the opportunity to learn from the error
- The health care organization's and individual provider's liability insurers
- Appropriate organization staff, including risk managers or quality assurance representatives
- Others who could provide emotional support or problem-solving help

Conferring with other members of the care team following an adverse event enables the provider to clarify factual details and the proper sequence of what occurred. It can also help to identify what needs to be done in response to the event.

A Joint Commission standard in the "Ethics, Rights, and Responsibilities" chapter of accreditation manuals indicates that the responsible licensed independent practitioner or his or her designee should inform the patient (and when appropriate, his or her family) about unanticipated outcomes of care, treatment, and services. This means that patients and, when appropriate, their families must be informed about the outcomes of care, including unanticipated outcomes such as sentinel events.

Good communication between providers and patients is instrumental in achieving positive care outcomes. Yet health care professionals often do not tell patients or families about their mistakes. Fear of malpractice litigation and the myth of perfect performance reinforce poor provider communication of errors to patients and their families. There is little doubt that the current malpractice crisis is a deterrent to the openness required for quality improvement.[6] However, errors not communicated to patients, families, fellow

Sample Medication Error Occurrence Report

Today's Date: _____ Reported By: _____

Completed By: _____

Initials of staff member filling medication: _____

Initials of staff member checking medication: _____

Date of incident: _____

Patient name: _____ Date of birth: _____

Location: _____

Circle all items that describe medication error occurrence:
1. Wrong medication
2. Incorrect dose of medication
3. Incorrect dosage form
4. Wrong patient
5. Incorrect label
6. Delivered to wrong patient
7. Clinical judgment error (for example, failure to properly evaluate drug interaction screen, approval of medication for use in a patient whose disease state contraindicates the use of the drug)

Explain: _____

Briefly describe the incident, outlining all known factual information:

_____

_____

Results of occurrence (circle all that apply):
1. Error discovered before medication taken
2. Medication taken: _____ Number of doses: _____
3. No apparent patient injury
4. Patient injury:

Explain: _____

_____

Change in process or education to avoid error from occurring in the future:

Figure 2-4. Unlike a general form or questionnaire, this sample medication error occurrence report exemplifies a form specific to medication errors.
Source: Lynn Moran, RPh, BS, Grove City, OH. Used with permission.

Sentinel Event Notification Checklist

SENTINEL EVENT
Occurrence: _____
Date and Time: _____
Contact Person: _____

Chief Executive Officer
Name: _____
Office Phone Number: _____
After-hours Phone Number: _____
Name/Phone of Designated Backup: _____
Notified by: _____
Date and Time: _____
Results of Contact: _____

Chief Nursing Officer
Name: _____
Office Phone Number: _____
After-hours Phone Number: _____
Notified by: _____
Date and Time: _____
Results of Contact: _____

Medical Staff Director
Name: _____
Office Phone Number: _____
After-hours Phone Number: _____
Notified by: _____
Date and Time: _____
Results of Contact: _____

Risk Manager
Name: _____
Office Phone Number: _____
After-hours Phone Number: _____
Notified by: _____
Date and Time: _____
Results of Contact: _____

Legal Counsel
Name: _____
Office Phone Number: _____
After-hours Phone Number: _____
Notified by: _____
Date and Time: _____
Results of Contact: _____

Public Relations Director
Name: _____
Office Phone Number: _____
After-hours Phone Number: _____
Notified by: _____
Date and Time: _____
Results of Contact: _____

Chair, Board of Directors
Name: _____
Office Phone Number: _____
After-hours Phone Number: _____
Notified by: _____
Date and Time: _____
Results of Contact: _____

Figure 2-5. This checklist can be used as a guide to properly notify the relevant officers following the occurrence of a sentinel event. Fill in the appropriate names and phone numbers and keep the information in a location readily accessible to managers and supervisors. The list should be periodically reviewed and updated.

Source: Adapted from Spath P.: Avoid panic by planning for sentinel events. *Hosp Peer Rev* 23(6):117, 1998. Used with permission.

Sidebar 2-1. Practical Issues for Physicians in Disclosing Medical Mistakes to Patients

Definition of a Medical Mistake

A medical mistake is a commission or an omission with potentially negative consequences for the patient that would have been judged incorrect by skilled and knowledgeable peers at the time it occurred.

Deciding Whether to Disclose a Mistake

In general, a physician has an obligation to disclose clear mistakes that cause significant harm that is remediable, mitigable, or compensable. In cases in which disclosing a mistake seems controversial, the decision should not be left to the individual physician's judgment.* It is important to obtain a second opinion to represent what a reasonable physician would do and be willing to defend in public. This second opinion is best obtained from an institution's ethics committee or quality review board rather than from informal consultation with peers.

Timing of Disclosure

Disclosure should be made as soon as possible after the mistake but at a time when the patient is physically and emotionally stable.

Who Should Disclose the Mistake?

When a mistake is made by a physician in training, responsibility is shared with the attending physician. It may be most appropriate for the attending and house officer to disclose the mistake to the patient together. When a mistake is made by a practicing physician, he or she should disclose the mistake to the patient. When the mistake results from the system of medical care delivery, it may be appropriate to involve an institutional representative in the disclosure, such as an administrator, risk manager, or quality assurance representative.

What to Say?

Disclosure is often difficult, for technical as well as emotional reasons. The facts of the case may be too complicated to be explained easily and may not be known precisely. The physician may be tempted to frame the disclosure in a way that obscures that a mistake was made. In telling the patient about an error, the physician should do the following:

- Treat it as an instance of breaking bad news to the patient.
- Begin by stating simply that he or she regrets that he or she has made a mistake or error.
- Describe the decisions that were made, including those in which the patient participated.
- Describe the course of events, using nontechnical language.
- State the nature of the mistake, consequences, and corrective action taken or to be undertaken.
- Express personal regret and apologize for the mistake.
- Elicit questions or concerns from the patient and address them.
- Ask if there is anyone else in the family to whom he or she should speak.

---

* A Joint Commission standard in the "Ethics, Rights, and Responsibilities" chapter states that the responsible licensed independent practitioner or his or her designee informs the patient (and when appropriate, his or her family) about the outcomes of care, treatment, and services, including unanticipated outcomes.

> **Sidebar 2-1. Practical Issues for Physicians in Disclosing Medical Mistakes to Patients,** *continued*
>
> **Consequences of Disclosure**
>
> Physicians are most often concerned about the potentially harmful consequences of disclosing a mistake—particularly the risk of a lawsuit. Serious mistakes may come to light even if the physician does not disclose them. Any perception that the physician tried to cover up a mistake might make patients angry and more litigious. The risks inherent in disclosing a mistake may be minimized if the following things happen:
>
> - Patients appreciate the physician's honesty.
> - Patients appreciate that physicians are fallible.
> - Disclosure is prompt and open.
> - Disclosure is made in a manner that diffuses patient anger.
> - Sincere apologies are made.
> - Charges for associated care are forgone.
> - A prompt and fair settlement is made out of court.
>
> **Disclosure of Mistakes Made by Other Physicians**
>
> A physician may encounter situations where he or she recognizes that a colleague physician has made a mistake. That colleague may choose to disclose the mistake or not. The physician recognizing the mistake has the following options:
>
> - Wait for the other physician to disclose the mistake.
> - Advise the other physician to disclose the mistake.
> - Simultaneously advise quality assurance or risk management.
> - Arrange a joint meeting to discuss the mistake.
> - Tell the patient directly of the error.
>
> The physician may be reluctant to disclose a colleague's error due to the following:
>
> - Lack of definitive information
> - Fear of hurting the colleague's feelings
> - Fear of straining a professional relationship
> - Fear of a libel suit
> - The sense that he or she could easily have made the same error ("There but for the grace of God go I")
> - Social norms against "tattling" on peers

Source: Adapted from McPhee S.J., et al.: Practical issues in disclosing medical mistakes to patients. Presented at the Examining Errors in Health Care Conference, Rancho Mirage, CA: Oct. 13–15, 1996.

staff members, and organizations are errors that do not contribute to systems improvement.

Disclosing mistakes to patients and their families is difficult, at best. Yet legal and ethical experts generally advise practitioners to disclose mistakes to patients and their families in as open, honest, and forthright a manner as possible. One suggestion is that physicians have an ethical duty to disclose errors when the adverse event does one of the following:

- Has a perceptible effect on the patient that was not discussed in advance as a known risk
- Necessitates a change in the patient's care

- Potentially poses an important risk to the patient's future health
- Involves providing a treatment or procedure without the patient's consent[7]

This idea maintains that disclosure of a mistake may foster learning by compelling the physician to acknowledge it truthfully and that the physician-patient relationship can be enhanced by honesty.[8] Disclosing a mistake might even reduce the risk of litigation, in fact, if the patient appreciates the physician's honesty and fallibility as a fellow human being. Another study reports that the risk of litigation nearly doubles when patients are not informed by their physicians of moderately serious mistakes.[9] Physician guidelines in disclosing medical mistakes to patients are offered by yet another report.[10] Sidebar 2-1, pages 45-46, outlines practical issues a physician may encounter in disclosing an error to a patient or his or her family. Please note that these are guidelines about issues to consider, not Joint Commission requirements. Organizations should be aware that the disclosure of an error or event requires individualized handling. Risk management or legal counsel should be involved in helping to guide communication with the patient and his or her family.

Onward with Root Cause Analysis

Having developed and implemented a sentinel event policy, the organization is now ready to start performing root cause analyses and developing an action plan. The next four chapters present in a step-by-step, workbook format how to perform a root cause analysis and develop, implement, and assess an improvement-driven action plan.

References

1. Croteau, Richard J.: Sentinel events, root cause analysis, and the trustee. *Trustee* 56(3):33–4, March 2003.
2. Perper J.A.: Life-threatening and fatal therapeutic misadventures. In Bogner M.S. (ed): *Human Error in Medicine*. Hillsdale, NJ: Lawrence Erlbaum Associates, 1994, p. 33.
3. Spath P.: Avoid panic by planning for sentinel events. *Hosp Peer Rev* 23(4):117, 1998.
4. Spath, p. 117.
5. Keyes C.: Responding to adverse events. *Forum* 18(1):2–3, 1997.
6. Blumenthal D.: Making medical errors into…"medical treasures". *JAMA* 272(23):1867–1868, 1994.
7. Cantor M., Barach P., Derse A., Maklan C., Schafer Wlody G., Fox E.: Disclosing Adverse Events to Patients. *Joint Commission Journal on Quality and Safety*, January 2005, Volume 31, Number 1.
8. Wu A.W., McPhee S.J.: Education and training: Needs and approaches for handling mistakes in medical training. Presented at the Examining Errors in Health Care Conference, Rancho Mirage, CA: Oct. 13–15, 1996.
9. Witman A.B., Hardin S.: Patients' responses to physicians' mistakes. *Forum* 18(4):4–5, 1997.
10. McPhee S.J., et al.: Practical issues in disclosing medical mistakes to patients. Presented at the Examining Errors in Health Care Conference, Rancho Mirage, CA: Oct. 13–15, 1996.

Chapter 3
Preparing for Root Cause Analysis

Step 1: Organize a Team

Step 2: Define the Problem

Step 3: Study the Problem

Step 4: Determine What Happened

Step 5: Identify Contributing Process Factors

Step 6: Identify Other Contributing Factors

Step 7: Measure—Collect and Assess Data on Proximate and Underlying Causes

Step 8: Design and Implement Interim Changes

Step 9: Identify Which Systems Are Involved—The Root Causes

Step 10: Prune the List of Root Causes

Step 11: Confirm Root Causes and Consider Their Interrelationships

Step 12: Explore and Identify Risk Reduction Strategies

Step 13: Formulate Improvement Actions

Step 14: Evaluate Proposed Improvement Actions

Step 15: Design Improvements

Step 16: Ensure Acceptability of the Action Plan

Step 17: Implement the Improvement Plan

Step 18: Develop Measures of Effectiveness and Ensure Their Success

Step 19: Evaluate Implementation of Improvement Efforts

Step 20: Take Additional Action

Step 21: Communicate the Results

This first workbook chapter describes how to prepare for a root cause analysis. It covers organizing a team, defining the problem, and studying the problem. The information is presented in a practical and user-friendly way. To help illustrate the steps of root cause analysis, sentinel events involving a suicide, elopement, medication error, and treatment delay are described as examples throughout this and subsequent chapters. A description of each sentinel event appears in Sidebar 3-1, pages 50-51. Checklists and worksheets are presented throughout the chapter. Use this and the following three chapters as a workbook—fill in the blanks.

A sentinel event or a near miss has occurred in an organization. Leadership has been informed and, in the case of an actual sentinel event, the organization has completed preliminary response procedures, including ensuring patient safety, risk containment, and prevention of repeat action (see Chapter 2). The appropriate staff members have documented the event and ensured communication with appropriate stakeholders.

Step One: Organize a Team

1 The first step involved in conducting a root cause analysis might be to assign a team to assess the sentinel event or potential sentinel event. Leaders must lay the groundwork by creating an environment conducive to root cause analysis and improvement through team initiatives. Often, leaders need to assure staff that organization improvement through the identification and reduction of risks, rather than the assignment of blame, is the objective. Guilt, remorse, fear, and anxiety are common emotions felt by staff following the occurrence of a sentinel

Sidebar 3-1. Sentinel Event Examples

Suicide
A 20-year-old male is admitted for observation to the behavioral health care unit of a general hospital. He has a well-documented history of depression. On his second day in the unit, he attends a particularly clamorous group session. Following the session, between 10:00 A.M. and 11:00 A.M., he commits suicide in his bathroom by hanging himself from the shower head with bedding sheets. A registered nurse finds him at 11:05 A.M., calls a code, and starts unsuccessful resuscitation efforts.

Elopement
Nursing staff in a long term care facility note that an 80-year-old woman with a history of progressive dementia is unusually irritable and restless. She is pacing, talking in a loud voice, and complaining about a number of issues. The nurses on duty are unable to appease her or to determine the cause of what they view as a bad mood. Staff members frequently remind the woman to move away from the exit door. In the evening, the staff discover that the woman is no longer on the unit, nor in the building. The woman left the facility without warm clothing on a cold evening with subzero temperatures. She is found dead the following morning in a wooded area near the facility. Death was caused by exposure.

Treatment Delay
A 60-year-old woman goes to an ambulatory health care organization to receive her annual physical from her long-time physician. The physician gives the woman a prescription for an annual mammogram, which she schedules for two weeks later. Following the mammogram, the woman is informed that she will hear from her physician's office. A week later, a nurse in the physician's office calls the woman and informs her that additional mammogram views are required. The nurse does not express the physician's wish that the tests be done immediately nor that there is a potential health problem. Required to perform extra duties because of short staffing, the nurse files the X-ray reports in the woman's medical record rather than in the proper file for tests requiring follow-up.

The woman does not forget the need for a follow-up mammogram and calls the physician's office to ascertain whether a repeat mammogram has been ordered. Another office employee assumes that if the woman did not get a call from the physician directly, the woman has nothing to worry about. The woman does not question the employee's answer, nor tell her about the nurse's call, and attempts to think no more about it.

Several weeks later, the woman calls the physician's office again, noting that she can feel a hard lump in her breast and mentioning that it hurts. The physician tells her to come into the office right away. Upon review of her record, the physician finds the results and orders another mammogram with needle localization "Stat." The woman has the test, which identifies a change in the size of a nodule from a previous mammogram. This requires an immediate biopsy, which is positive. Subsequent surgery reveals that the cancer has metastasized.

> ## Sidebar 3-1. Sentinel Event Examples, *continued*
>
> **Medication Error**
>
> A 60-year-old man receiving home care services complains about a headache to his home health nurse on each of the nurse's three visits during a one-week period. The man indicates that he is tired of bothering his primary care physician about various symptoms. At the conclusion of the third visit, the nurse offers to discuss the man's complaint with his primary care physician upon return to the agency. When the nurse discusses the headache with the man's physician, the physician instructs the nurse to call the local pharmacy with the following prescription:
>
> > Fioricet Tabs. #30
> > Sig: 1-2 tabs q 4-6 hours prn headache
> > Refill x3
>
> In error, the nurse telephones the pharmacy and provides the following prescription:
>
> > Fiorinal Tabs. #30
> > Sig: 1-2 tabs q 4-6 hours prn headache
> > Refill x3
>
> The man has a long history of peptic ulcer disease, which resulted in several hospitalizations for gastrointestinal bleeding. The man began taking the Fiorinal, which contains 325mg aspirin per tablet. In contrast, the intended medication—Fioricet—contains 325mg acetaminophen per tablet.
>
> The man completes the entire first prescription and 15 tablets of the first refill. At this point, he goes to the emergency department with acute abdominal pain, blood in the stool, and a hemoglobin of 4.9. He is immediately admitted to the intensive care unit. Within hours, he needs life support. After several units of blood and a four-week hospital stay, the man recovers and is able to return to his home following this "near miss" sentinel event.

event. These emotions must be addressed and discussed at the earliest stages of team formation. Leaders must put staff members at ease so that staff members can contribute to risk reduction. Leaders further lay the groundwork by empowering the team to make changes or recommendations for changes, providing the resources (including time to do the work), and ensuring a defined structure and process for moving forward. *See* Checklist 3-1, page 52.

What Is a Team?

Webster's dictionary defines the word *team* as a number of individuals associated with one another. Team implies a group that is dynamic and working together toward a well-defined goal. In the health care environment, a team should be interdisciplinary. Unlike committees that meet for a long period of time for an ongoing purpose, a team generally meets on an ad hoc basis for shorter periods of time. After a specific

> ## Checklist 3-1.
> ## Essential Elements for a Team Go-ahead
>
> While developing a team and selecting team members, ensure that the following three elements are present in the organization's leadership:
>
> ☐ Awareness of and support from top leadership
> ☐ Leadership commitment to provide necessary resources, including time
> ☐ An empowered team with authority and responsibility to recommend and implement process changes

project is completed, the team often disbands—with a sense of accomplishment.

Why Use a Team?
A team approach brings increased creativity, knowledge, and experience to solving a problem. Just as a patient's care is provided by a team, the analysis of that care should be carried out by a team including representatives of all the professional disciplines involved in that care. Multidisciplinary teams distribute leadership and decision making to all levels of an organization. Teams in health care organizations provide a powerful way to integrate services across the continuum of care.[1] They also provide a powerful and often successful way to effect systemwide improvement.

Who Should Work on the Team?
A team may be established on an ad hoc basis, or, if the relevant disciplines or services are represented, the core of an appropriate team may already exist in the form of a targeted performance improvement team or some other type of team. The selection of team members is critical. The team should include staff at all levels closest to the issues involved—those with fundamental knowledge of the particular process involved. These individuals are likely to be those with the most to gain from improvement initiatives. The team may include the individual(s) directly involved in the sentinel event if the organization chooses to include them. The decision about whether to include the individual(s) directly involved in the sentinel event can be made on a case-by-case basis. For instance, if an individual is traumatized by the event, it may make sense to instead invite another person of the same discipline with comparable process knowledge to join the team. Later, during the action planning stage when systems and processes are being redesigned, it may make sense to bring individuals directly involved with the sentinel event onto the team so that they feel they have made a positive contribution to the change process. The team should also include an individual with some distance from the process, but who possesses excellent analytical skills. The team should also include at least one individual with decision-making authority as well as individuals critical to the implementation of anticipated changes. Team members should bring to the table a diverse mix of knowledge bases and should be knowledgeable about and committed to performance improvement. *See* Checklist 3-2, page 53.

Physician participation on performance improvement teams is vital. Improvement initiatives resulting from root cause analyses often address some aspect of clinical care. As a result, medical staff involvement is essential. Leaders should understand the barriers to physician involvement and take steps to overcome those barriers, which include skepticism about the purpose of root cause analyses and improvement teams, skepticism about relevance and effectiveness of teams, and lack of time and incentive to participate.

Organizations may also wish to think "outside the box" in terms of possible team members. Might a former patient, family member, or other community member be able to provide a unique perspective and valuable input? For example, perhaps the town's retired pharmacist or a former patient that experienced a "near miss" sentinel event could be invited to join the root cause analysis team. If one of the suspected root causes of a sentinel event relates to information management, perhaps a member of the local chapter of an information management association or organization could be invited.

Team composition may need to change as the team moves in and out of areas within the organization that affect or are affected by the issues being analyzed. An organization should allow for and expect this to happen. However, the core team members should remain as stable as possible throughout the process, at least in terms of leadership and areas or functions represented. Realistically, the selection of all team members cannot take place until the broad aim of the improvement initiatives to be generated by the root cause analysis and improvement action plan are identified.[2]

For example, to investigate the root cause of a medical gas utility disruption that led to the death of a patient when his oxygen supply was inadvertently cut off, the core team should include physicians, representatives from clinical staff (nursing and/or respiratory therapy), management, administration, and information management; someone who works primarily with medical gases and the utility management program; and if vendors are a primary part of the analysis, someone from the purchasing or contracting services department. A description of possible members of teams examining the sentinel events described in Sidebar 3-1 follows.

The core team investigating the **suicide** in a behavioral health care unit might include the following individuals: a nurse(s) from the behavioral health unit; an occupational therapist, physical therapist, or recreation therapist (who has clinical skills and knowledge, but would not necessarily spend much time on the behavioral health care unit); a social worker on the

> **Checklist 3-2.**
> **Team Composition**
>
> While drawing up a tentative list of team members, check to ensure that the team includes
>
> ☐ Individuals closest to the event or issues involved
> ☐ Individuals critical to implementation of potential changes
> ☐ A leader with a broad knowledge base, who is respected and credible
> ☐ Someone with decision-making authority
> ☐ Individuals with diverse knowledge bases

unit; a representative from the education department; a psychiatrist (who attended the patient); a medical staff leader who understands processes and has the authority to change medical staff policy; the manager of the behavioral health unit; a representative from quality improvement or risk management (who will act as the facilitator); an administrative representative at the vice-president level (such as nursing, patient care, or an associate VP) who can make changes; a safety engineer; and a safety consultant (on ad hoc basis).

The core team investigating the **elopement** of a resident from a long term care facility might include the following individuals: the director of nursing, a unit nurse (regular care provider), a nursing assistant (who regularly cared for the resident), the medical director, the safety director or person responsible for the safety program, the individual responsible for performance improvement (facilitator of the group), a social service worker, and a unit activity staff member.

The core team investigating the **treatment delay** in an ambulatory care organization might include the following individuals: the director of the ambulatory care organization, a staff physician, the medical director, the appointments scheduler, a staff nurse, the staff educator, the office manager, the manager of the laboratory used by the organization, the pharmacy supplier used by the organization, and the director or manager of quality/performance improvement.

The core team investigating the **medication error** in a home health agency might include the following individuals: a home health nurse, a nursing supervisor, an agency director or administrator, a member of the pharmacy supplier's staff, a local pharmacist (ad hoc), the medical director, the quality/performance improvement coordinator, and an information technology or management staff member, as available.

To have a significant effect in a health care organization, performance improvement must address clinical care. The participation of physicians and other medical staff members on root cause analysis and improvement teams is critical. Leaders must understand the barriers to medical staff involvement and take steps to overcome those barriers.[3]

The team should have a leader who is knowledgeable, interested, and skilled at group consensus building and applying the tools of root cause analysis. This person guides the team through the root cause analysis process while encouraging open communication and broad participation. The leader may function as a facilitator, or a separate team member can be assigned to play the facilitator role. This individual should be skilled at being objective and moving the team along. It is best if the leader and facilitator are not stakeholders in the processes and systems being evaluated. Ad hoc members who can provide administrative support, additional insight, and resources should be identified as well. Use Worksheet 3-1, page 68, to indicate proposed team members.

At the first team meeting, the leader should establish ground rules that will help the team avoid distractions and detours on the route to improvement. The following ground rules provide a framework that will allow the team to function smoothly:

- *Team mission:* The leader should establish the group's mission or focus as one of systems improvement rather than individual fault finding.
- *Sentinel event policy:* The leader should provide copies of the sentinel event policy and procedures, enabling all team members to become familiar with expectations.
- *Decision making:* The group must decide what kind of consensus or majority is needed for a decision, recognizing that decisions belong to the entire team.
- *Attendance:* Attendance is crucial. Constant late arrivals and absences can sabotage the team's efforts. Set guidelines for attendance.
- *Meeting schedule:* For high attendance and steady progress, the team should agree on a regular time, day, and place for meetings. These matters should be revisited at various times during the team's life.
- *Timeline:* The leader should present a timeline at the initial meeting to keep the group on track as it moves toward its quality improvement goals.
- *Opportunity to speak:* By agreeing at the outset to give all members an opportunity to contribute and to be heard with respect, the team will focus its attention on the important area of open communication.
- *Disagreements:* Similarly, the team must agree to disagree. It must acknowledge and accept that members will openly debate differences in viewpoint. Discussions may overflow outside the meeting room, but members should feel free to say in a meeting what they say in the hallway.

Tip: Team Size
Core teams limited in size to fewer than 10 individuals tend to perform with greater efficiency. Experts needed at different points can be added as ad hoc team members and attend only the relevant meetings.

> ## Sidebar 3-2. Leadership Techniques for Promoting High-Quality Group Discussion
>
> The following techniques for leaders can help to ensure high-quality group discussion:
>
> - Use small groups to report ideas.
> - Offer quiet time for thinking.
> - Ask each person to offer an idea before allowing comments or second turns at speaking.
> - Keep the discussion focused on observations rather than opinions, evaluations, or judgments.
> - Keep the discussion moving forward within the allotted time frame.
> - Pull the group together if the discussion fragments into multiple conversations.
> - Encourage input from quiet members.
> - Prevent domination by one group member.
> - Ensure consensus or group decisions.

- *Assignments:* The team should agree to complete assignments within the particular time limits so that delayed work from an individual does not delay the group.
- *Other rules:* The team should discuss all other rules that members feel are important. These can include whether senior management staff can drop in, whether pocket pagers should be checked at the door, what the break frequency is, and so forth.

See Sidebar 3-2, above, for techniques team leaders or facilitators can use to ensure high-quality group discussion.

Step Two: Define the Problem

One of the first steps taken by the root cause analysis team is to define the problem—that is, to describe, as accurately as possible, what happened or what nearly happened. The purpose of defining the problem as clearly and specifically as possible is to help focus the team's analysis and improvement efforts. If the team defines and understands the problem clearly, much time, effort, and frustration can be saved.

Tool: *Brainstorming*

In response to a sentinel event, the team might ask, "What actually happened or what alerted the staff to a 'near miss'?" Initially, the problem or event can be defined simply, such as the following:
- Surgery was performed on the incorrect site.
- Patient committed suicide by hanging.
- Patient died following overdose of drug.
- Abductor tried to leave the unit with an infant that did not belong to him/her.

These simple statements focus on what happened or the outcome, not on why it happened. During later steps in the root cause analysis process, the team will focus on the sequence of events, on the *whys*, and on contributing factors.

For "near misses" or improvement opportunities, the preceding problem statements could be restated as follows:
- Surgery was almost performed on the incorrect site.
- Patient attempted to commit suicide by hanging.
- Patient received overdose of drug but survived without long-term consequences.

> **Tip: Criteria for a Well-Defined Problem**
> A well-defined problem statement states what is wrong and focuses on the outcome, not why the outcome occurred.

- Abductor was discovered by nurse before leaving the unit.

Use Worksheet 3-2, page 69, to define the problem.

Particularly in the event of a "near miss," multiple problems may be present. Which problem should be selected first for analysis? Each team needs to develop ranking criteria to help meet this challenge. One option is to rank problems by their cost impact, organization priority, consequence or severity, safety impact, or real or potential hazard.[4] Problems should be addressed one at a time. The highest-ranked problem should be tackled and solved before initiating work on lower-ranked problems. This topic will be explored in more depth in Chapter 6.

Tool: Multivoting

Help with Problem Definition

The information disseminated from the Joint Commission's Sentinel Event Database can be helpful in an organization's identification of a problem or area for analysis. The purpose of this database is to increase general knowledge about sentinel events, their causes, and strategies for prevention. The Joint Commission collects and analyzes data from the review of actual sentinel events, root cause analyses, action plans, and follow-up activities in all types of health care organizations. By sharing the lessons learned with other health care organizations, the hope is that the risk of future sentinel events will be reduced. Organizations can learn about sentinel events that occur with significant frequency, their root causes, and possible risk reduction strategies through the Joint Commission's publication *Sentinel Event Alert* (*see* Sidebar 3-3, right) and the newsletter *Joint Commission Perspectives*® received by the CEO of every accredited organization. All organizations can use the areas or problems outlined here as a starting point in the identification of a problem area for

---

Sidebar 3-3. Sentinel Event Alert

The following topics have been covered in the Joint Commission's *Sentinel Event Alert* publication:

- Patient controlled analgesia by proxy (Dec. 2004)
- Preventing, and managing the impact of, anesthesia awareness (Oct. 2004)
- Revised guidance to prevent kernicterus (Aug. 2004)
- Preventing infant death and injury during delivery (Jul. 2004)
- Preventing surgical fires (Jun. 2003)
- Infection control related sentinel events (Jan. 2003)
- Bedrail-related entrapment deaths (Sep. 2002)
- Prevention of treatment delays (June 2002)
- Prevention of ventilator-related deaths and injuries (Feb. 2002)
- Prevention of wrong-site surgery (Dec. 2001 and Aug. 1998)
- Prevention of medication errors (Sep. 2001, May 2001, Feb. 2001, Nov. 1999, Feb. 1998)
- Prevention of needlestick and sharps injuries (Aug. 2001)
- Prevention of medical gas mix-ups (Jul. 2001)
- Prevention of exposure to Cruetzfeldt-Jakob disease (June 2001)
- Prevention of fires in the home care setting (Mar. 2001)
- Prevention of adverse events related to infusion pumps (Nov. 2000)
- Prevention of falls (Jul. 2000)
- Prevention of operative and postoperative complications (Feb. 2000)
- Prevention of blood transfusion errors (Aug. 1999)
- Prevention of infant abductions (Apr. 1999)
- Prevention of restraint deaths (Nov. 1998)
- Prevention of inpatient suicides (Nov. 1998)

Current and past issues of *Sentinel Event Alert* can be found on the Joint Commission's Web site at http://www.jcaho.org/about+us/news+letters/sentinel+event+alert/index.htm.

analysis. Table 3-1, page 58, lists the sentinel events most frequently reviewed by the Joint Commission. Sentinel events reported in the national media can also serve as a source of ideas for problem analysis.

Identification of risk points can often yield a helpful problem list. *Risk points* are those specific places in a process or system that are susceptible to failure or system breakdown. They generally result from a flaw in the initial design of the process or system, a high degree of dependence on communication, nonstandardized processes or systems, and failure or absence of backup.

For example, risk points during the medication-use process include interpretation of an illegible order by a pharmacist and the time during which a registered nurse mixes the medication dose to administer to a patient. In surgical procedures requiring the use of lasers, a risk point occurs during the use of anesthetic gases, which, if not properly synchronized with use of the laser, can ignite and cause fires. During preoperative procedures, verification of the body side and site constitutes a risk point.

Tool: Brainstorming

Identification of failure-prone systems yields problem areas requiring focus through root cause analysis. A number of factors increase the risk of system failures, including complexity—a high number of steps and hand-offs in work processes. Complex systems may be dynamic, with constant change and tight time pressure and constraints. The tight coupling of process steps can increase the risk of failure. Tightly coupled systems or processes do not provide much slack or the opportunity for recovery. Sequences do not vary, and delays in one step throw off the entire process. Variable input and process steps that are nonstandardized can also increase the risk of process failure, so can processes carried out in a hierarchical rather than team structure.

For example, medication ordering is frequently cited as a risk-prone system due to organization hierarchies. Nurses and pharmacists may be reluctant to question physicians writing the orders. Some organization cultures, in fact, may create a hierarchical rather than team structure for the entire medication-use process. Similarly, verification of surgical sites by surgical team members can suffer from hierarchical pressures. Nurses may be reluctant to question physicians. Language barriers coupled with a hierarchical culture can present a particularly dangerous scenario. Worksheet 3-3, page 70, can be used to identify risk-prone systems in an organization.

Most frequently, sentinel events result from multiple system failures. They also frequently occur at the point where one system overlaps or hands off to another. An organization should be tracking high-risk, high-volume, and problem-prone processes as part of its performance improvement efforts. High-risk, high-volume, problem-prone areas vary by organization and are integrally related to the care, treatment, and services provided. For example, to reduce the risk of infant abductions, a large maternity unit should focus on its infant-parent identification process. To reduce the risk of patient suicide, a behavioral health care unit should focus on its suicide risk assessment process. The list of frequently occurring sentinel events published by the Joint Commission (*see* Table 3-1, page 58), an organization's risk management data, morbidity and mortality data, performance data (including sentinel event indicators and aggregate data indicators), or information about problematic processes generated by field-specific or professional organizations can provide starting places to find such processes.

Tool: Brainstorming

Developing a Preliminary Work Plan and Reporting Mechanism

After a team has chosen a problem for analysis and defined the problem, it can develop a preliminary work

Table 3-1. Types of Sentinel Events Reviewed by the Joint Commission

Since establishing its Sentinel Event Database in 1995, the Joint Commission has tracked the frequency of occurrence of various types of sentinel events. The following events appear most frequently in the database:

- Patient suicide
- Wrong-site surgery
- Operative or postoperative complications
- Medication error
- Delay in treatment
- Patient fall resulting in injury or death
- Patient death or injury in restraints
- Assault, rape, or homicide
- Transfusion error
- Perinatal death/loss of function
- Patient elopement resulting in injury or death
- Infection-related event resulting in injury or death
- Fire
- Anesthesia-related event resulting in injury or death
- Ventilator death/injury
- Maternal death
- Medical equipment–related event resulting in injury or death
- Abduction of any individual receiving care, treatment, or services
- Discharge of an infant to the wrong family
- Utility systems–related event resulting in injury or death

---

plan for investigating the sentinel event through root cause analysis. The plan should outline the overall strategy, key steps, individuals responsible for each step, target dates, and reporting mechanisms.

To develop the overall strategy, a team can articulate what it is trying to accomplish. This is the *aim statement*. An aim statement can be sharpened[5] by completing the sentences found in Worksheet 3-4, page 71. A specific aim statement answers the question, "What are we trying to accomplish?" It should be objective and measurable. Possible aim statements for the investigation of each sample sentinel event described in Sidebar 3-1, pages 50-51, follow.

The aim statement for the **suicide** investigation might read as follows:

> Our aim is to improve the quality of suicide risk assessment on admission. The process begins when the individual served is admitted to the behavioral health care unit (or, it might begin in an emergency department, therapist's office, and so forth *before* the individual is admitted) and ends with an appropriate assessment of suicide risk and the individual's placement at the appropriate level of care. By working on this process, we expect to enhance the effectiveness of suicide risk assessment and achieve appropriate risk assessments with 98% to 100% of our admissions. We must work on this process to reduce the risk of patient suicide.

The aim statement for the **elopement** investigation might read as follows:

> Our aim is to improve the quality of assessment of residents for possible risk for elopement. The process begins with the initial assessment of at-risk status when the resident is admitted to the facility, continues through regular reassessment during the resident's stay, and ends only when the resident is discharged from the facility or passes away. By working on this process, we expect to enhance the effectiveness of initial risk assessment and achieve

ongoing risk reassessment with 99% to 100% of our residents. We must work on this process to reduce the risk of resident elopement.

The aim statement for the **treatment delay** investigation might read as follows:

> Our aim is to improve processes that reduce the risk of sentinel events associated with treatment delays. The processes must include a leadership definition of appropriate staffing levels and the provision of high-quality initial orientation for staff members. The processes also include regular assessment of ongoing staff competence and ongoing assessment of staffing needs. By working on these processes, we expect to enhance the effectiveness of initial orientation and ongoing competence assessment with 90% to 100% of staff members achieving assessment scores of 90% or higher on all post-training tests. We must work on this process to reduce the risk of treatment delays associated with insufficient staff orientation and training or insufficient staffing.

The aim statement for the **medication error** investigation might read as follows:

> Our aim is to improve the effective communication of information related to medication orders. The process begins when the home health care nurse consults with the physician regarding a medication and ends with the accurate administration of the right drug to the right individual, in the right dosage, at the right time, with the right frequency, using the right administration technique, and via the right route. By improving the process for communicating critical medication-related information, we expect to enhance the accuracy and timeliness of medications administered by our nurses to home care patients and therefore decrease adverse medication occurrences by 10% in each of the next five years. We must work on this process to reduce the likelihood of injury or death due to medication errors.

The creation of a detailed work plan is critical to the process and to securing management support. A plan outlining target dates for accomplishing specific objectives provides a tool against which to guide and measure the team's progress.

The full work plan should include target dates for major milestones and key activities in the root cause analysis process. These can mirror the steps of the root cause analysis and action plan itself, including the following:
- Defining the event and identifying the proximate and underlying causes
- Collecting and assessing data about proximate and underlying causes
- Designing and implementing interim changes
- Identifying the root causes
- Planning improvement
- Testing, implementing, and measuring the success of improvements

Checklist 3-3, page 60, indicates the key steps to include in a work plan for a root cause analysis. Each activity is described further in later chapters. Use Worksheet 3-5, page 72, to outline key steps, individuals responsible, and target dates for a root cause analysis. Also outline the reporting mechanisms and use the checklist portions to double-check overall strategy and report quality.

Tool: Gantt chart

A team's outline of the reporting mechanism aims to ensure that the right people receive the right information at the right time. At the beginning of the process, the team leader or facilitator should establish a means of communicating team progress and findings to senior leadership. Keeping senior leaders informed on a regular basis is critical to management support of the root cause analysis initiative and implementation of its recommendations. Although it is difficult to provide guidelines on how "a regular basis" should be

Checklist 3-3. Key Steps in Root Cause Analysis and Improvement Planning

The work plan can include the following key activities with target dates for each major milestone:

☐ Organize a team Completion date: _____

☐ Define the problem Completion date: _____
    ☐ Choose area(s) for analysis
    ☐ Develop a plan

☐ Study the problem Completion date: _____
    ☐ Gather information

☐ Determine what happened and why (proximate causes) Completion date: _____
    ☐ Identify process problem(s)
    ☐ Determine which patient care processes are involved
    ☐ Determine factors closest to the event
    ☐ Extract measurement data

☐ Identify root causes Completion date: _____
    ☐ Determine which systems are involved

☐ Design and implement an action plan for improvement
    ☐ Identify risk reduction strategies Completion date: _____
        ☐ Formulate actions for improvement
        (considering actions, measures, responsible
        party, desired completion date, and so forth)
        ☐ Consider the impact of the improvement action
    ☐ Design improvements Completion date: _____
    ☐ Implement action plan Completion date: _____
    ☐ Measure effectiveness Completion date: _____
        ☐ Develop measures of effectiveness
        ☐ Assure success of measurement
    ☐ Evaluate implementation efforts Completion date: _____
    ☐ Communicate results Completion date: _____

Note: In preparing a root cause analysis in response to a sentinel event that is reviewable by the Joint Commission, remember that the analysis must be completed no more than 45 days after the event's occurrence or becoming aware of the event.

defined, because this varies widely depending on circumstances, communication with senior leaders should increase in frequency with the following:
- Serious adverse outcomes
- Repeated adverse events
- Events requiring solutions from multiple parts of the organization
- Possible solutions requiring the investment of significant amounts of money
- The media's involvement in the case and its solutions

Frequency of communication also varies according to the actions required in the short term to prevent recurrence of the event. Communication frequency should be weighed against the speed with which information emerges from the investigation. If information is emerging rapidly, the team leader should give thought to the most productive timing for communication. A description of reporting considerations for each of the sample root cause analysis investigations follows.

The reporting mechanism for the **suicide** investigation should ensure that the psychiatrist on the team is providing his or her colleagues with regular updates on the team's progress at clinical department meetings. This prepares the medical staff for recommended policy changes. Similarly, at executive staff meetings, the vice president on the team should be providing the CEO, chief operating officer, and other leaders with regular updates on the team's progress. Communication should be frequent to foster leadership acceptance of future recommendations, particularly those involving significant resources.

The reporting mechanism for the **elopement** investigation should ensure that the safety director is providing the facility management and operations staff with regular updates on the team's progress. This prepares them for any recommended building alterations to enhance the safety of the care environment.

The reporting mechanism for the **treatment delay** investigation in an ambulatory care organization should ensure that the office manager is keeping the physician/medical director informed of the team's progress on a regular basis. This prepares the medical director for any changes that might be warranted with respect to staffing levels and staff orientation, training, and ongoing competence assessment.

The reporting mechanism for the **medication error** investigation should ensure that the information technology staff member is keeping his or her colleagues informed of the team's progress. This facilitates the smooth integration of any new processes or technology that may be recommended to enhance safe medication ordering.

Step Three: Study the Problem

The team is now ready to start studying the problem. This involves collecting information surrounding the event or "near miss." Time is of the essence because key facts can be forgotten in a matter of days. In fact, the individual(s) closest to the event or "near miss" may have already collected some information that the team can use as a starting point. Often a written statement provided by individuals involved in the event and prepared as near the time of the event as possible can be useful throughout the root cause analysis process. At times, the individual(s) closest to the event may withhold critical information due to the fear of blame. The team should consider how to eliminate such fear. It may be necessary in some instances to obtain the individual's written statement and then proceed without his or her contribution in the early stages of the analysis.

Early on, the team should give thought to how information is to be recorded. Some methods are more suitable than others. For example, audiotaping or videotaping an interview with someone intimately involved with the event is likely to increase the individual's defensiveness. Note taking is an effective way to record interviews. Videotapes, drawings, and/or photographs are also effective media to record physical

> **Sidebar 3-4.**
> **Ways to Record Information**
>
> The following media can be used to record information obtained during a root cause analysis:
>
> - Written notes
> - Audiotapes
> - Photographs or drawings
> - Videotapes
>
> It is important that the team obtains legal counsel on how to protect the information from discovery.

evidence. For instance, if an organization experienced an accidental death when an individual served was strangled after slipping through guard rails on a bed, a videotape or photo of the bed with guard rails in place provides evidence of the position of the device following the event. The team should not rely on the memory of anyone. Instead, complete notes, audiotapes, videotapes, photographs, and drawings ensure accuracy and thoroughness of information collection. In addition, they aid in reporting the team's progress. *See* Sidebar 3-4, above, for ways of recording information.

In all cases, the team should seek guidance from the organization's legal counsel regarding protection of information from discovery through its inclusion in peer review and other means. The team should also seek guidance from the organization's ethics committee concerning patient confidentiality and the information collected during the root cause analysis (*see* Chapter 2, pages 37-47).

The team must ensure focus of information or data collection. Collecting a huge amount of information, much of which might not be related in any way, is both unproductive and confusing. To focus collection efforts, examine the problem statement and collect data along potential lines of inquiry. Figure 1-2, page 16, can provide guidance for potential lines of inquiry. For example, if a problem statement such as, "Patient jumped from unsecured window," suggests an environment of care or human resources problem, collect data relevant to training, security systems, and so forth. A sampling of information that might be collected relevant to the suicide, elopement, treatment delay, and medication error examples described in Sidebar 3-1, pages 50-51, follows:

Information to be collected in the **suicide** investigation might include an environment of care inventory of all fixtures in the behavioral health care units, and data on which fixtures are *breakaway compliant* and which are not. That is, those that are or are not capable of breaking automatically in response to a predetermined external force (for example, the weight of an individual).

Information to be collected in the **elopement** investigation might include an environment of care inventory of unattended or unmonitored exits; availability and functionality of wander-prevention technology, such as electric bracelets and wired exits; data related to the thoroughness and frequency of initial resident assessment and ongoing reassessment for elopement risk; and information regarding how data about individuals at risk for elopement are integrated into initial and ongoing care plans.

Information to be collected in the **treatment delay** investigation might include data about how test results are processed within the organization and how staff is trained in these processes initially and on a continuing basis. Data related to competence assessment testing and staffing levels would also be valuable.

Information to be collected in the **medication error** investigation might include data on how medication orders are transmitted to local pharmacies and the percentage of queries and errors due to illegible physician handwriting, misinterpretation of physician handwriting, telephone or verbal orders, and order transcription. Data related to the frequency of nurse communication about a new medication and patient education efforts would also be valuable.

While information or data collection occurs throughout the root cause analysis process, the team may also want to gather three key types of information at this early stage:
1. Witness statements and observations from those closest to the event (or potential event), as well as those indirectly involved
2. Physical evidence related to the event (or potential event)
3. Documentary evidence[6]

Each type of information is fully addressed in the following section.

Witness Statements and Observations

Interviews with staff members can provide a wealth of information during a number of stages of root cause analysis. Closely following an event or "near miss," interviews with staff members *directly* involved can probe for what happened or almost happened and why (proximate causes). Interviews with staff members *indirectly* involved can explore possible root causes. Later in the process, interviews can provide insight into possible improvement initiatives and implementation strategies.

Conducting interviews is both an art and a science. Some people do it well; some do not. The team should carefully consider who is best suited to interview each subject and the best possible timing and sequence of interviews to be conducted. The goal of the interviews is to identify facts, possible systemic causes, and improvement opportunities—*not* to place blame. The team should identify all likely interview candidates at each stage and be aware that people tend to forget information or remember it incorrectly, rationalize situations, and perceive situations differently.

Four discrete stages of what normally appears to be a continuous interview process are preparing for the interview, opening the interview, conducting the interview, and closing the interview.[7] The following descriptions are adapted from *The Root Cause Analysis Handbook*.

When **preparing for the interview**, the interviewer plans the interview. This involves reviewing previously collected information, developing carefully worded interview questions that are open-ended, scheduling the interview, determining how information will be recorded and documented, preparing to answer questions that the interviewee is likely to raise, identifying material that should be available as a reference during the interview, and establishing the physical setting. Carefully worded responses to such questions as, "Why do you want to talk with me?" and "What will you do with the information I provide?" can go a long way toward reducing the interviewee's defensiveness, and so can a neutral setting where privacy is ensured and interruptions avoided.

When **opening the interview**, the interviewer should greet the interviewee, exchange informal conversation,

---

Tip: Overcoming Interviewee Defensiveness

- Restate the focus and purpose of the interview and reiterate that information obtained will be used to help prevent future occurrences of an adverse event, rather than to fix blame.
- Send positive, supportive messages through statements such as, "What you've said is so helpful," and "I understand, and you've obviously given this a lot of thought."
- Gently ask about a defensive reaction and probe why the interviewee feels threatened. (Take great care here to ensure that this will not do more harm than good.)

> ## Sidebar 3-5.
> ## Types of Open-ended Questions
>
> Open-ended questions ensure that the interviewee provides more than a simple yes or no answer. Three types of open-ended questions that can be used effectively to gain the depth and breadth of information needed during interviews follow.
>
> **Exploratory Questions**
> Exploratory questions can be used effectively to begin the discussion or a new topic. They encourage the interviewee to provide both comprehensive and in-depth information. Examples are
>
> - "What can you tell me about … ?"
> - "What can you recall about … ?"
>
> **Follow-up Questions**
> Often, it may be necessary to clarify or amplify information provided by the interviewee. Follow-up questions can help. Examples are
>
> - "What do you mean by … ?"
> - "Can you tell me more about … ?"
> - "What is … ?"
> - "How did this come about?"
>
> **Comment Questions**
> Comment questions (or statements) encourage elaboration and express interest while not sounding like a question. Examples are
>
> - "Can you tell me more about that?"
> - "Could you please describe that further?"

Source: Adapted from Ammerman M.: *The Root Cause Analysis Handbook: A Simplified Approach to Identifying, Correcting, and Reporting Workplace Errors.* New York: Quality Resources, 1998, pp. 53–54.

state the purpose of the interview, and answer the interviewee's questions. The goal is to establish rapport, put the interviewee at ease, establish credibility, and get the interviewee involved in the interview process as quickly as possible. The interviewer should indicate the amount of time required for the interview so that the interviewee knows what to expect.

When **conducting the interview**, the interviewer poses his or her open-ended questions. Open-ended questions elicit information by encouraging more than a "yes" or "no" response. In contrast, leading questions put words in the interviewee's mouth (for example, "This was only a minor problem, wasn't it?"). There are a number of different ways to pose such questions and a variety of question types to ensure that the questions sound natural, several of which are shown in Sidebar 3-5, left.

A two-step probing technique, using an exploratory question and then a follow-up question asking "why," can yield valuable information (for example, the sequence of "What can you tell me about the administration of restraints in the unit?" followed by "Why do you think this is the case?"). This technique should be reserved for important areas because its repetition could make the interviewee feel "drilled."

Throughout the interview, the interviewer should listen well, avoid interrupting the subject, avoid talking excessively, ask purposeful questions, and summarize throughout the interview to ensure a proper understanding of what the subject has related. The interviewer should also be aware of his or her own body language, as well as of the interviewee's body language and other nonverbal cues.

When **closing the interview**, the interviewer should check to ensure that he or she has obtained all necessary information; ask the interviewee if he or she has any questions or concerns; summarize the complete interview to ensure that the information accurately reflects the interviewee's words; and thank the interviewee, expressing appreciation for his or her time, honesty, and assistance.

After the interviewee leaves the interview area, the interviewer should document any further observations and identify follow-up items. Conclusions and results should be communicated to the root cause analysis team, as appropriate.

Group interviews can be more efficient than individual interviews, but disadvantages should be considered and weighed with care. Disadvantages include dominance by more vocal members of the group and the emergence of groupthink, which can stifle individual accounts of an event.

When in-person interviews are not possible, telephone interviews can provide an alternative. However, the telephone has some serious limitations. It is much more difficult to establish and maintain rapport when eye contact is not part of the equation, and, of course, nonverbal cues are much harder to read. Written responses from an observer to specific questions raised by the team are another alternative (*see* Worksheet 3-6, pages 73-76). However, this means is less likely than either in-person or telephone interviews to elicit in-depth information. A matter as seemingly trivial as how much space is provided for answers on the form can have a significant impact on the quantity of information provided. In addition, when the observer must put something in writing, his or her concern about the privacy and confidentiality of the information may increase defensiveness, thereby preventing full disclosure and honesty.

Remember the following points when gathering information from caregivers:
- People's memories and their willingness to help can be affected by the way questions are asked
- Interviewees should be informed that follow-up interviews are a normal part of the root cause analysis process and do not reflect any suspicion of the information provided in initial interviews
- Interviewees should be encouraged to contact the team leader with any concerns or additional information[8]

Physical Evidence

Physical evidence related to the event or "near miss" should be gathered at an early stage. As described in Chapter 2, page 40, preserving the evidence immediately following the event or near miss can be essential to understanding why an event occurred or almost occurred. In many instances, physical evidence inadvertently (or deliberately) may be taken, misplaced, destroyed, moved, or altered in some way.

Interviews with personnel closest to the event can help the team identify relevant physical evidence including equipment, materials, and devices. Physical evidence for a sentinel event involving a medication error, for example, might include the drug vial, syringe, prescription, IV drip, filter straws, and medication storage area. Physical evidence for a suicide in a 24-hour care setting might include breakaway bars and fixtures in the shower or elsewhere, a window, a ceiling, and other sites. Physical evidence for a wrong-site surgery might include the X-rays, the operative arena, surgical instruments, and so forth.

The evidence should be thoroughly inspected by a knowledgeable team member, ad hoc member, or consultant. Perhaps equipment was not fully assembled or parts were missing. Observations from the inspection should be documented. All physical evidence should be labeled with information on the source, location, date and time collected, basic content, and name of the individual collecting it and then secured in a separate area, if feasible. If not, such as with a large piece of equipment, the item should be tagged to indicate that it failed and that its use is prohibited, pending investigation results.

Documentary Evidence

Documentary evidence includes all material in paper or electronic format that is relevant to the event or possible event. This could include the following:

- Patient records, physician orders, medication profiles, laboratory test results, and all other documents used to record patient status and care
- Policies and procedures, correspondence, and meeting minutes
- Human resource-related documents such as performance evaluations, competence assessments, and physician profiles
- Indicator data used to measure performance
- Maintenance information such as work orders, equipment logs, instructions for use, vendor manuals, and testing and inspection records

All such evidence should be examined, secured, and labeled appropriately.

Documentary evidence varies considerably, based on the actual sentinel event or possible sentinel event. Examples of documentary evidence for various error types follow. This information is a starting place in considering the kind of documentary evidence needed for any organization's root cause analysis.

For a **medication error** involving the administration of the wrong medication and the subsequent death of a patient, documentary evidence could include the following:
- The patient's medical record
- Trending data on medication errors
- Procedures for drug-allergy interaction checking
- Pharmacy lot number logs
- Pharmacy recall procedure
- Maintenance logs for equipment repair
- Downtime logs for computer software
- Equipment procedure logs for mixing of solutions;
- The error report to the US Pharmacopoeia and state licensing agency
- Lab test results of drug samples
- Interdepartmental and interorganization memos or reports regarding the event

For a **mechanical error** involving the shut-off of oxygen and the subsequent death of a patient, documentary evidence could include the following:

- Procedures for informing patient care areas about downtime of mechanical or life support systems
- Construction and technical documents and drawings of the medical gas distribution system
- Inspection, performance measurement, and testing policies and procedures
- Policies and procedures for shut-off of utility systems
- Utility system performance measurement data
- Documents related to the utility systems planning process
- Management competence assessment programs
- Technical staff training, retraining, and competence assessment programs in utilities systems processes
- Incident and emergency reporting procedures
- Maintenance procedures and logs

For a **suicide**, documentary evidence could include the following:
- The patient's history and physical on admission
- Staff observation notes
- Attendance logs for unit activities
- Policies and procedures for patient observation
- An inventory of items in the patient's possession on admission
- The patient's psychosocial assessment
- All physician and nursing notes prior to the incident.

Literature Review

At this point and throughout the root cause analysis, a thorough review of the professional literature is an important component of the root cause analysis process. Literature searches can yield helpful information about the event at hand and other organizations' experiences with a similar event. Literature can help identify possible root causes and improvement strategies. Appropriate associations and societies can provide a good starting point in the review process. Obtain a variety of information on the subject. A review of other organizations' practices and experiences can help avoid mistakes and inspire creative thinking. Information that might be obtained to investigate causes and improvement strategies for the sample sentinel events includes the following:

For a **suicide** event, the team might obtain suicide risk assessment policies, procedures, and forms from other organizations. A team member might conduct an online literature search to obtain suicide risk assessment protocols from relevant professional journals.

For an **elopement** event, the team might obtain resident assessment policies, procedures, and forms from other long term care organizations and, specifically, information related to how they assess at-risk-for-elopement status. The facility or safety manager might obtain information from other organizations related to systems used to ensure appropriate security in the environment of care, such as wander-prevention technology. Assessment protocols from relevant professional journals might be helpful as well.

For a **treatment delay** event, the team might obtain policies, procedures, and protocols for communicating abnormal test findings from the professional literature and peer ambulatory care organizations. Training and competence assessment literature could also provide insight for improvement strategies. Professional organizations might be a source of information on criteria for calling in additional specialists.

For a **medication error** event, the team might contact other home care organizations to obtain information about the policies and protocols used to ensure a safe medication-use process. An online literature review could provide improvement strategies recommended by other health care organizations following a sentinel event or near miss.

Tools to Use

The team should begin to consider performance measurement tools that might be helpful in the next step of the root cause analysis—searching for proximate causes and determining what happened and why. Information can be collected on such tools as brainstorming, flowcharts, cause-and-effect diagrams, Pareto charts, scatter diagrams, affinity diagrams, bar graphs, line graphs, pie graphs, Gantt charts, and timelines.

Tools: *Brainstorming, flowcharts, cause-and-effect diagrams, Pareto charts, scatter diagrams, affinity diagrams, bar graphs, line graphs, pie graphs, Gantt charts, timelines*

References

1. Phillips K.M.: *The Power of Health Care Teams: Strategies for Success*. Oakbrook Terrace, IL: Joint Commission on Accreditation of Healthcare Organizations, 1997, pp. 18, 30.
2. Nelson E.C., Batalden P.B., Ryer J.C. (eds): *Clinical Improvement Action Guide*. Oakbrook Terrace, IL: Joint Commission on Accreditation of Healthcare Organizations, 1998, p. 27.
3. Phillips, p. 43.
4. Wilson P.F., Dell L.D., Anderson G.F.: *Root Cause Analysis: A Tool for Total Quality Management*. Milwaukee, WI: ASQC Quality Press, 1993, pp. 39-40.
5. Nelson, et al., pp. 34–35.
6. Spath P.L.: *Investigating Sentinel Events: How to Find and Resolve Root Causes: A Simplified Approach to Identifying, Correcting, and Reporting Workplace Errors*. Forest Grove, OR: Brown-Spath & Associates, 1997, pp. 50–52.
7. Ammerman M.: *The Root Cause Analysis Handbook*. New York: Quality Resources, 1998, pp. 49–61.
8. Spath, p. 51.

Worksheet 3-1. Composing the Team

Fill in the team leader, facilitator (if necessary), and team members, including ad hoc members who serve on an as-needed basis. Ensure interdisciplinary representation by including information such as job titles, degrees, and responsibilities.

Core Team Members

1. Leader _____
2. Facilitator _____
3. _____
4. _____
5. _____
6. _____
7. _____
8. _____
9. _____
10. _____

Ad Hoc Members

_____
_____
_____
_____
_____
_____

Worksheet 3-2. Defining the Problem

Use this space to formulate a simple, one-sentence definition of the event or "near miss."

A sentinel event occurred: What happened?

_____

_____

_____

_____

_____

_____

_____

_____

A "near miss" occurred: What nearly happened?

_____

_____

_____

_____

_____

_____

_____

_____

Worksheet 3-3. Identifying Risk-Prone Systems

Use this worksheet to identify risk-prone systems within your organization.

Systems involving variable input include

_____

_____

Complex systems include

_____

_____

Nonstandardized systems include

_____

_____

Tightly coupled systems include

_____

_____

Systems with tight time constraints include

_____

_____

Systems with a hierarchical, nonteam structure include

_____

_____

Worksheet 3-4. Sharpening an Aim Statement

1. The organization's aim is to improve the quality and value of (fill in the name of the care process):

   _____
   _____
   _____
   _____.

2. This process starts with _____
   _____

   and ends when_____
   _____.

3. By working on this process, the team expects that (fill in the anticipated better and measurable outcomes)

   _____
   _____
   _____
   _____.

4. It is important to work on this process now because (insert reasons that make this important)

   _____
   _____
   _____
   _____.

Worksheet 3-5. Preliminary Planning

Overall strategy

☐ Does it include the team's aim? ☐ Is it objective? ☐ Is it measurable?

Key steps/initiatives	**Individual responsible**	**Target date**

Reporting mechanisms

Who receives copies of the reports?

_____

_____

_____

_____

_____

Are the reports or other output from the team

☐ Informative? ☐ Accurate? ☐ Timely?

Worksheet 3-6. Gathering Information

Use the following worksheet as a place to start gathering written information from individuals who cannot be interviewed in person or by telephone. Be aware that the amount of space you provide for each question often determines the amount of information provided by the respondent. If a detailed answer to a certain question is desired, be sure to leave plenty of space and provide a prompt such as, "Please provide as much information as possible."

What conditions existed prior to the event?

_____

_____

_____

_____

_____

_____

What procedures or processes were being conducted prior to and during the event?

_____

_____

_____

_____

_____

_____

Worksheet 3-6. Gathering Information, *continued*

Who was present and involved in the event?

_____
_____
_____
_____
_____
_____
_____

What indicated that a problem was occurring?

_____
_____
_____
_____
_____
_____
_____

How did you respond?

_____
_____
_____
_____
_____

Worksheet 3-6. Gathering Information, *continued*

How did others in the area respond? What procedures or processes might have been associated with the event?

_____
_____
_____
_____
_____
_____
_____

What might have caused the event?

_____
_____
_____
_____
_____
_____

Worksheet 3-6. Gathering Information, *continued*

How might the event be prevented in the future?

_____
_____
_____
_____
_____
_____
_____
_____
_____

Any other comments or thoughts?

_____
_____
_____
_____
_____
_____
_____
_____
_____

Chapter 4

Determining What Happened and Why: The Search for Proximate Causes

Step 1: Organize a Team

Step 2: Define the Problem

Step 3: Study the Problem

Step 4: Determine What Happened

Step 5: Identify Contributing Process Factors

Step 6: Identify Other Contributing Factors

Step 7: Measure—Collect and Assess Data on Proximate and Underlying Causes

Step 8: Design and Implement Interim Changes

Step 9: Identify Which Systems Are Involved—The Root Causes

Step 10: Prune the List of Root Causes

Step 11: Confirm Root Causes and Consider Their Interrelationships

Step 12: Explore and Identify Risk Reduction Strategies

Step 13: Formulate Improvement Actions

Step 14: Evaluate Proposed Improvement Actions

Step 15: Design Improvements

Step 16: Ensure Acceptability of the Action Plan

Step 17: Implement the Improvement Plan

Step 18: Develop Measures of Effectiveness and Ensure Their Success

Step 19: Evaluate Implementation of Improvement Efforts

Step 20: Take Additional Action

Step 21: Communicate the Results

This chapter provides guidance on how a team can search for proximate or direct causes. It represents the first level of probing to determine in more detail what happened, or nearly happened, and why. The team must also look at process and other contributing factors. This chapter also provides information on choosing what to measure and analyze further so that the team can determine root causes and an effective improvement plan. Figure 1-3, pages 20-23, from Chapter 1, provides the framework for this and subsequent steps of root cause analysis.

4 Step Four: Determine What Happened

Prior to this point in the process, the team has created a very simple, one-sentence definition of what happened or could have happened. The next step involves creating a more detailed description or definition of the event. This description provides the *when, where,* and *how* details of the event. It should include the following:
- A brief description of what happened
- Mention of where and when the event occurred (place, date, day of week, and time)
- Identification of the area or services affected by the event

For example, with a sentinel event involving the death of a patient in restraints, a more detailed definition of the event might state, "Death of an 18-year-old male from burns and smoke inhalation following a fire started by the patient with matches in a room in Unit E where the patient was restrained. Event occurred on Friday, January 1 at 11 A.M." The relevant areas for this sentinel event might be nursing, medicine, security, and physical plant. *See* Worksheet 4-1, page 88, for questions to ask in developing a detailed definition of an event.

In creating this more detailed definition of an event, team members should be careful not to jump to conclusions concerning what happened prior to completing the root cause analysis. For example, perhaps the team's problem statement at this point reads, "80-year-old female found in room beside her bed, lying on floor dead. Event occurred sometime between 0200 and 0330, Thursday, March 4." Did the patient die because of the fall? Or, did the patient fall after or while dying? A root cause analysis will help the team identify the cause of death. In this example, relevant areas or services affected by the event might include nursing (to investigate monitoring systems and medication administration), biomedical (to investigate the type of bed, alarm, and call light system), staffing office (to investigate whether the type of staff—regular or float—impacted the event), education (to investigate orientation and training provided to staff and patient), pharmacy (to investigate patient medications), and medical staff protocols (to investigate medications ordered for the patient).

It is often helpful to determine the sequence of events by developing a timeline or flowchart. These tools can help the team retain focus on the facts of the event. Ensure that the source of each fact is noted on the tool so the source can be consulted if more information is needed.

Tools: *Flowchart, timeline*

5 Step Five: Identify Contributing Process Factors

Root cause analysis involves repeatedly asking "Why?" to identify the underlying root causes of an event or possible event. At this point, the team asks the first of a series of "why" questions. The goal of the first "why" question is to identify the proximate causes of the event. *Proximate* or *direct causes* are the most apparent or immediate reasons for an event. They involve factors lying closest to the origin of an event, and they can generally be gleaned by asking, "Why did the event happen?" As mentioned in Chapter 1 (page 8), a proximate cause typically involves a special-cause variation. Special-cause variation is not inherently present in a process. It is intermittent and unpredictable. If the team is measuring a process using a control chart, special-cause variation appears as those points outside the control limits. In contrast, common-cause variation appears as points between the control limits.

Tool: *Control chart*

In most cases, identifying the proximate causes is simple; in other cases, it might take some digging. For example, in the restraint-related death, proximate or direct causes could include "missed observation" and "patient possessed contraband matches." In the case of the patient found dead by her bed, proximate causes could include "failure to monitor patient," "bed alarm not working," "call light not working," "patient not properly oriented to use of call light," "incorrect sedation dispensed," or "incorrect administration of sedation."

Underlying causes of proximate causes in the health care environment may relate to the provision of care or to other processes. Hence, identification of the patient care processes or activities involved in the sentinel event or potential sentinel event will help the team identify contributing causes. At this point, asking and answering the following three questions will assist the team:

1. Which processes were involved in the event or almost led to an event?
2. What are the steps and linkages between the steps in the process as designed, as routinely performed, and as occurred with the sentinel event?
3. Which steps and linkages were involved in, or contributed to, the event?

A variety of tools can help ensure a thorough response to these questions. A flowchart is a useful way to visualize the response to "What are the steps in the process?" Brainstorming can be used to identify processes and supplement the list of process steps to ensure that all relevant steps are included. Cause-and-effect diagrams, change analysis, and failure mode and effects analysis (FMEA) are useful techniques in analyzing a response to "Which steps and linkages were involved in or contributed to the event?"

Tools: *Brainstorming, flowchart, cause-and-effect diagram, change analysis, FMEA*

The team can then probe further by asking three more questions:
1. What is currently done to prevent failure at this step or its link with the next step?
2. What is currently done to protect against a bad outcome if there is failure at this step or linkage?
3. What other areas or services are affected?

Comparing the flowchart of the process as designed and specified in written policies and procedures to the flowcharts of the process as routinely performed or as occurring with the sentinel event can alert the team to staff actions that circumvent policies and procedures either knowingly or unknowingly. Staff members who perform the processes in question should routinely compare their actual actions to the prescribed policies and procedures to detect any discrepancies.

In addition to identifying discrepancies between actual actions and the prescribed policies and procedures, however, the organization needs to know whether the current systems and processes produce the expected outcomes. In many organizations, policies and procedures are written in response to regulatory requirements or adverse outcomes and then forgotten—and never evaluated for effectiveness. Instead, the policies should be routinely evaluated for their effectiveness. In addition, many policies and procedures contain too much information, making compliance onerous and, therefore, less likely.

Fault tree analysis can be used to study current failure prevention activities. Barrier analysis can be helpful in looking at what is currently done to protect against a bad outcome if there is a failure. FMEA can be a useful tool in examining other affected areas or services. Use Worksheet 4-2, page 89, as a summary of questions to raise and tools to consider using.

Tools: *Fault tree analysis, barrier analysis, FMEA*

Step Six: Identify Other Contributing Factors

In the health care environment, proximate causes tend to fall into a number of distinct categories beyond, and in addition to, process factors. These include the following:
- Human factors
- Equipment factors
- Controllable or uncontrollable environmental factors
- Other factors

To identify the proximate cause of an event involving human factors, the team might ask, "What human factors were relevant to the outcome?"

To identify the proximate cause of an event involving equipment factors, the team might ask, "How did the equipment performance affect the outcome?" To identify the proximate cause of an event involving environmental factors, the team might ask, "What

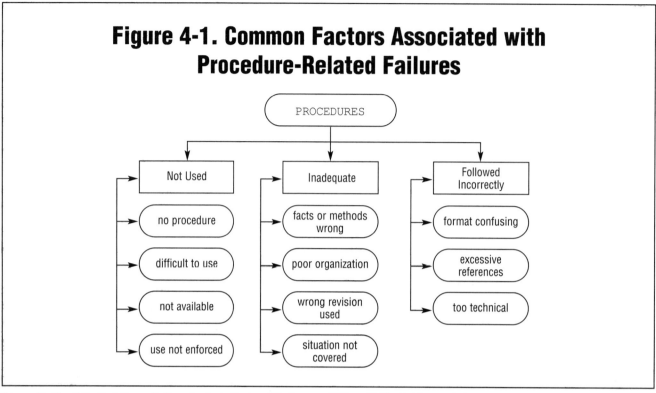

Source: Mobley R.K.: *Root Cause Failure Analysis*. Boston, MA: Newnes, 1999, p. 40. Used with permission.

factors directly affected the outcome? Were such factors within or truly beyond the organization's control?"

Finally, the team might ask, "Are there any other factors that have directly influenced this outcome?" Figures 4-1 through 4-3, pages 80-81, identify common factors associated with procedure-, training-, and equipment-related failures. Use Worksheet 4-3, pages 90-91, to identify factors closest to the event.

Continuing the example involving the death of a patient in restraints following a fire, the team might conclude that proximate causes included the following:
- Human factors involving failure to follow observation procedures, failure to implement contraband checking procedures, and lack of de-escalation training
- Assessment factors involving failure of the safety or patient assessment tools or incomplete patient assessment; assessment beyond scope of staff (for example, completed in the emergency department by staff with no behavioral health assessment competence)
- Environmental factors involving difficulty in conducting regular patient observations due to design of space
- Controllable equipment factors involving failure of smoke detector

Similarly, in identifying the proximate causes for a suicide, a team might conclude that proximate causes include the following:
- Human factors involving failure to follow policies on precaution orders or failure to conduct appropriate staff education/training
- Assessment process factors involving a faulty initial assessment process that did not include identification of past history of suicide attempts or an immediate psychiatric consultation
- Process or human factors involving a faulty history and physical assessment that did not identify patient suicide risk factors
- Equipment factors involving a nonfunctional paging system that delayed communication with the patient's physician

Determining What Happened and Why: The Search for Proximate Causes **Chapter 4**

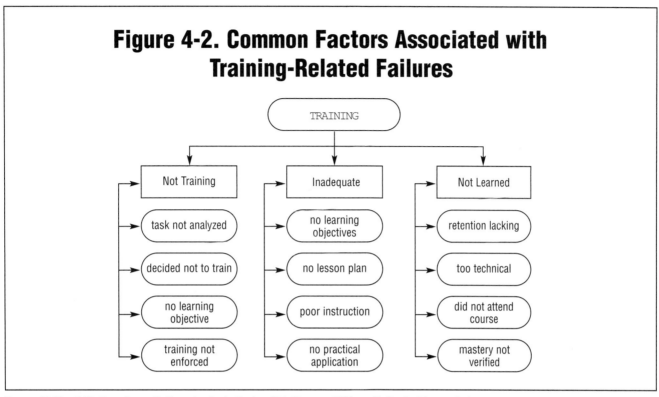

Source: Mobley R.K.: *Root Cause Failure Analysis*. Boston, MA: Newnes, 1999, p. 41. Used with permission.

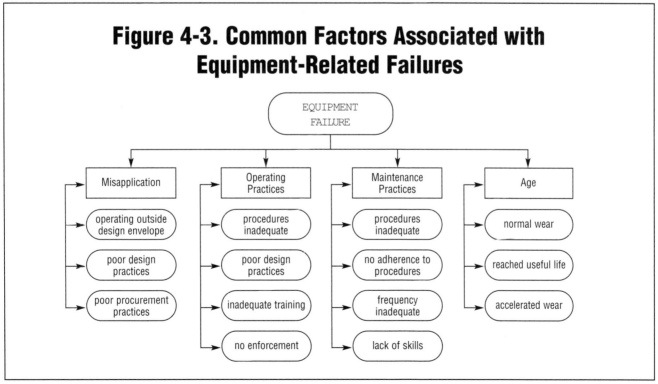

Source: Mobley R.K.: *Root Cause Failure Analysis*. Boston, MA: Newnes, 1999, p. 38. Used with permission.

Brainstorming to identify all possible or potential contributing causes may be a useful technique for teams at this stage of the root cause analysis. Following traditional brainstorming ground rules, such as not labeling anything a bad idea, and ensuring that team members do not express reactions or provide commentary as ideas are expressed, is critical to success. The focus must be on improving patient outcomes rather than individual performance. Affinity diagrams can be used to help sort or organize the causes or potential causes into natural, related groupings. Cause-and-effect diagrams can help highlight the numerous factors involved in an event.

Tools: Brainstorming, affinity diagram, cause-and-effect diagram

While asking questions to uncover causes, the team leader should keep team members focused on processes, not people. By repeatedly asking "Why?" the team can continue working until it feels it has exhausted all possible questions and causes. The importance of this stage cannot be overstated. It provides the initial substance for the root cause analysis without which a team cannot proceed.

After sorting and analyzing the cause list, the team may begin determining which process or system each cause is a part of and whether the cause is a special or common cause in that process or system. This process, described fully in the next chapter, helps to unearth system-based root causes.

Step Seven: Measure—Collect and Assess Data on Proximate and Underlying Causes

Data gathering must begin as soon as possible after the event occurs to prevent loss or alteration of the data. Data from people are the most easily altered or destroyed and need to be made a priority. Other forms of data are more stable; however, physical data need to be identified quickly to prevent their inadvertent loss or destruction.

To advance further toward discovering root causes, the team must explore in depth proximate and underlying causes. This exploration involves measurement—collecting and assessing relevant data. While this exploration is presented here as Step Seven, data collection and analysis initiatives may occur throughout root cause analysis and need not be sequential or follow Step Six and precede Step Eight.

Measurement is the process of collecting and aggregating data. The process helps assess the level of performance, determine whether improvement actions are necessary, and ascertain whether improvement has occurred.

The first purpose of measurement is to provide a baseline when little objective evidence exists about a process. For example, a health care organization may want to learn more about the current level of staff competence. A dementia long term care or psychiatric special care unit may want to know more about the effectiveness of the bed alarm systems to prevent patient falls and elopement. Specific indicators for a particular outcome or a particular step in a process may be used for ongoing data collection. When assessed, these data can help management and staff determine whether a process is ineffective and needs more intensive analysis. Data about costs, including costs of faulty or ineffective processes, may also be of significant interest to leaders and can be part of ongoing performance measurement.

The second purpose of measurement, more the focus here, is to gain more information about a process chosen for assessment and improvement. For example, perhaps a performance rate varies significantly from the previous year, from shift to shift, or from the statistical average. A team may be measuring staff compliance with the organization's restraint policy, for instance. Records may indicate that the staff on duty during weekend hours does not properly document the monitoring of patients in restraint or obtain appropriate orders for restraint use. Or, perhaps the data indicate that restraints are used with an increased frequency when specific personnel are present. Perhaps monitoring problems or inappropriate restraint use is suspected as part of a root cause of a sentinel event. Such findings may cause a health care organization to focus on a given process to determine opportunities for improvement. The target for further study is usually time limited and can test a specific population, a specific diagnosis, a specific service provided, or an organization management issue. Detailed measurement is then necessary to gather data about exactly how the process performs and about factors affecting that performance.

The third purpose of measurement is to determine the effectiveness of improvement actions. For example, a nursing unit that begins to use a new piece of equipment needs to establish a baseline performance rate and continue to measure use. Measurement can also demonstrate that key processes (for example, the preparation and administration of medications) are in control. When a process has been stabilized at an acceptable level of performance, it may be measured periodically to verify that the improvement has been sustained. Measurement to monitor improvement actions is described fully in Chapter 6.

In summary, data are collected to monitor the stability of existing processes, identify opportunities for improvement, identify changes that lead to improvement, and maintain changes.

Choosing what to measure is absolutely critical at all stages of root cause analysis—in probing for root causes and in assessing whether a recommended change or action represents an actual improvement (*see* Sidebar 4-1, right). Measurement requires indicators that are stable, consistent, understandable, easy to use, and reliable. *Indicators* or *performance measures* are devices or tools for quantifying the level of performance that actually occurs. They are valid if they identify events that merit review, and they are reliable if they accurately and completely identify occurrences (*see* Sidebar 4-2, page 84).

Sidebar 4-1. Choosing What to Measure

Choosing what to measure is extremely important. An organization may wish to start by defining the broad processes or systems most likely to underlie proximate causes. For example, if a team is investigating a medication error involving the process used to communicate an order to the pharmacy and the process used by pharmacy staff to check the dosage ordered, the team may decide to measure the following for a defined period of time:

- Time elapsed between when an order is written by medical staff and when the pharmacy receives the order by fax, pickup, or phone
- Time elapsed between when the dosage is checked by pharmacy staff and when medication is dispensed
- Time elapsed between when medication is dispensed and when medication is administered

---

Examples of an outcome indicator are "catheter-related sepsis for patients with a central venous access device" or "percentage of patients at risk for falls who actually experience falls while in the health care organization." An example of a process indicator is "patients older than 65 years of age having medication monitoring for drugs that can decrease renal function."

The two broadest types of indicators are *sentinel event indicators* and *aggregate data indicators*. A sentinel event indicator identifies an individual event or

> ## Sidebar 4-2. Definition of an Indicator or Measure
>
> An indicator (or measure) can be described in the following ways:
> - Quantitative—It is expressed in units of measurement.
> - Valid—It identifies events that merit review.
> - Reliable—It accurately and completely identifies occurrences.
> - A measure of a process or outcome—It involves a goal-directed series of activities or the results of performance.

phenomenon that is significant enough to trigger further investigation each time it occurs. Such indicators are well known in risk management. They help ensure that each event is promptly evaluated to prevent future occurrences. As required by Joint Commission performance improvement requirements, all health care organizations must monitor the performance of processes that involve risks or may result in sentinel events.

Although sentinel event indicators are useful to ensure patient safety, they are less useful in measuring the overall level of performance in an organization. In contrast, an aggregate data indicator quantifies a process or outcome related to many cases. Unlike a sentinel event, an event identified by an aggregate data indicator may occur frequently. Aggregate data indicators are divided into two groups, *rate-based indicators* and *continuous variable indicators*.

Rate-Based Indicators

Rate-based indicators express the proportion of the number of occurrences to the entire group within which the occurrence could take place, as in the following examples:

$$\frac{\text{Patients receiving cesarean sections}}{\text{All patients who deliver}}$$

$$\frac{\text{Total number of elopements}}{\text{Patients at risk for elopement (wandering and confused)}}$$

$$\frac{\text{Patients with central line catheter infections}}{\text{All patients with central line access devices}}$$

$$\frac{\text{Patient falls associated with adverse drug reactions}}{\text{All patient falls}}$$

The rate can also express a ratio comparing the occurrences identified with a different, but related phenomenon, as in the following example:

$$\frac{\text{Patients with central line infections}}{\text{Central line days}}$$

Continuous Variable Indicators

This type of aggregate data indicator measures performance along a continuous scale. For example, a continuous variable indicator might show the precise weight in kilograms of a patient receiving total parenteral nutrition (TPN). Or, it might record the number of written pharmacist recommendations accepted by the attending physicians. While a rate-based indicator might relate the number of patients approaching goal weights to the total number of patients on TPN, a continuous variable indicator measures the patient's average weight change (that is, the patient's weight one month minus the patient's weight the previous month).

See Checklist 4-1, page 85, for criteria that will help the team ensure that the measure or indicator selected is actually appropriate for monitoring performance. See Sidebar 4-3, page 85, for key questions the team should ask about measurement throughout the root cause analysis process.

Checklist 4-1. Criteria to Ensure Appropriate Data Collection

Choosing what to measure is critical, and so is ensuring that the data collected are appropriate to the desired measurement. The following checklist includes criteria to help the team ensure that the data collected are appropriate for monitoring performance:
- ☐ The measure can identify the events it was intended to identify
- ☐ The measure has a documented numerator and has a denominator statement or description of the population to which the measure is applicable
- ☐ The measure has defined data elements and allowable values
- ☐ The measure can detect changes in performance over time
- ☐ The measure allows for comparison over time within the organization or between the organization and other entities
- ☐ The data intended for collection are available
- ☐ Results can be reported in a way that is useful to the organization and other interested customers

Sidebar 4-3. Key Questions About Measurement

Throughout the root cause analysis, the team should ask the following questions concerning measurement:
- What will be measured? (This defines what is critical to determining root causes.)
- Why will this be measured? (This verifies the criticality of what will be measured.)
- What can be gained from such measurement? (This describes the incentives of measurement.)
- Who will perform the measurement?
- How frequent is the measuring?
- How will the data be used when measurement is completed?
- Is the measure or measurement reliable?
- Is measurement a one-time event or periodic process?
- What resources are needed for measurement? What is available?
- Do the measures consider dimensions of performance?

Additional information on measurement, including how to measure the effectiveness of improvement initiatives and assure the success of measurement, appears in Chapter 6.

8 Step Eight: Design and Implement Interim Changes

Even at this early stage, when the team has identified only proximate causes, some quick or immediate fixes may be appropriate. For example, in the case of an organization that experienced the suicide of a patient who was not identified as being at risk for suicide, the organization could immediately evaluate its current risk assessment tool to learn whether it meets current standards of practice. Or, it could start conducting mandatory in-service training for all staff on suicide risk assessment. Or the organization could place all patients with psychiatric or substance abuse diagnoses on suicide precautions. Or, the organization could address environment of care issues such as nonbreakaway shower heads and bed linens. In addition, the organization could evaluate the suicide risk assessment tool and the process used to check for contraband, and initiate meetings with the medical staff to discuss revisions to requirements for

Figure 4-4. Steps to Identify and Eliminate Proximate Causes of a Patient Suicide

ACTIVITY	3rd Qtr 2004			4th Qtr 2004			1st Qtr 2005			2nd Qtr 2005		
	Jul	Aug	Sep	Oct	Nov	Dec	Jan	Feb	Mar	Apr	May	Jun
Establish review team												
Expanded security rounds to include helipad												
Revised Suicide Precaution Policy												
Staff training: Suicide Precaution Policy												
Staff training: Assessment and interventions for patients with mental health needs												
Staff training: Patients leaving unit unattended												
Team meetings to assess plan-do-study-act (PDSA)												
Medical record review of all suicide precaution charts												
Concurrent assessment of patients on suicide precautions												

histories and physicals. A Gantt chart used by one organization to outline the key steps and time frames for a plan to eliminate proximate causes that led to a patient suicide appears as Figure 4-4, above.

 Tool: Gantt chart

In the case of an organization that experienced a wrong-site surgery, the organization could require a second staff member to observe operating room team procedures to assess compliance with the Universal Protocol for Preventing Wrong Site, Wrong Procedure, Wrong Person Surgery™.

Teams conducting root cause analysis need not wait until they finish their analysis to begin designing and implementing changes. During the process of asking "Why?" potential interventions emerge. Intermediate changes may not only be appropriate but necessary. First, they may be needed to reduce an immediate risk. For example, an unsecured window may need to be repaired and secured; an intoxicated employee should be removed from the environment immediately; and broken or malfunctioning equipment should be removed from the area of care, treatment, or service and secured. Second, they may also uncover additional causes that were previously masked but are critical to the search for the root cause. Finally, intermediate changes can be part of a plan-do-study-act (PDSA) cycle to test process redesign before implementing it organizationwide. For instance, an organization may wish to test the use of new bathroom hardware in one room before changing hardware organizationwide.

The process of sorting through reasons for the root cause has been called *identifying the web of causation*. "The key point is to identify the web of causation and to intervene on as many levels as possible in this web. It is important to recognize that the deeper one progresses in the chain or web of causation, the closer one gets to underlying, structural (root) causes."[1] Hence, although the team may make intermediate improvements along the way, it should not stop the root cause analysis process before the root cause is identified and corrective action is taken. Where intermediate actions are planned, the team should identify the following:

- *Who* is responsible for implementation
- *When* the actions will be implemented—including any pilot testing
- *How* the effectiveness of the actions will be evaluated

Again, however worthy short-term solutions may be, the organization must not stop after implementing these, but rather continue probing more deeply to arrive at the root causes and possible long-term solutions. Chapter 5 addresses how the team can continue this effort.

Reference

1. Altman D.G.: Strategies for community health intervention: Promises, paradoxes, pitfalls. *Psychosom Med* 57(3):226–233, 1995.

Worksheet 4-1. Further Defining What Happened

In developing a more detailed definition of what happened, the team should consider the following three questions:

1. What are the details of the event? Write a brief, two- or three-sentence description.

_____
_____
_____
_____
_____
_____

2. When and where did the event occur (place, date, day of week, and time)?

_____
_____
_____
_____
_____

3. What area(s) or service(s) was impacted?

_____
_____
_____
_____
_____
_____

Worksheet 4-2. Identifying Proximate Causes

To determine proximate causes of a sentinel event or possible sentinel event involving patient care or organization processes, the team can ask the following questions and consider using the following tools to aid in answering each question.

1. Which processes were involved or could have been involved in the event or "near miss?"
   Tools: ☐ Brainstorming   ☐ Cause-and-effect diagram

   _____
   _____

2. What are the steps in the process, as designed?
   Tools: ☐ Flowchart   ☐ Brainstorming

   _____
   _____

3. Which steps were (or could have been) involved in, or contributed to, the event or "near miss?"
   Tools: ☐ Cause-and-effect diagram   ☐ Change analysis   ☐ FMEA

   _____
   _____

4. What is currently done to prevent failure at this step?
   Tools: ☐ Fault tree analysis   ☐ Flowchart

   _____
   _____

5. What is currently done to protect against a negative outcome if there is failure at this step?
   Tool: ☐ Barrier analysis

   _____
   _____

6. What other areas or services are affected?
   Tools: ☐ Failure mode and effects analysis   ☐ Brainstorming

   _____
   _____

Worksheet 4-3. Identifying Factors Close to the Event

Use this worksheet to identify factors closest to the event or possible event.

Human factors included or could include

_____
_____
_____
_____
_____
_____

Equipment factors included or could include

_____
_____
_____
_____
_____
_____

Controllable environmental factors included or could include

_____
_____
_____
_____
_____
_____

Worksheet 4-3. Identifying Factors Close to the Event, *continued*

Uncontrollable environmental factors included or could include

_____
_____
_____
_____
_____
_____

Other factors included or could include

_____
_____
_____
_____
_____
_____

Chapter 5
Identifying Root Causes

This chapter addresses how a team identifies and validates the root causes of a sentinel event or "near miss." This represents a deeper level of digging to determine the systemic roots of a problem. Root causes are the most fundamental causal factors of an event. As such, their origin lies in common-cause variation of organization systems. (A discussion of variation can be found in Chapter 1, page 8.) Getting to the root cause of a sentinel event or "near miss" takes a lot of time and effort. It involves asking "Why?" until root causes are identified and then exploring the ramifications of each response. This chapter provides guidance on how to conduct such an exploration. Figure 1-3, pages 20-23, in Chapter 1 provides the framework for this and subsequent steps of the root cause analysis.

Step 1: Organize a Team
Step 2: Define the Problem
Step 3: Study the Problem
Step 4: Determine What Happened
Step 5: Identify Contributing Process Factors
Step 6: Identify Other Contributing Factors
Step 7: Measure—Collect and Assess Data on Proximate and Underlying Causes
Step 8: Design and Implement Interim Changes
Step 9: Identify Which Systems Are Involved—The Root Causes
Step 10: Prune the List of Root Causes
Step 11: Confirm Root Causes and Consider Their Interrelationships
Step 12: Explore and Identify Risk Reduction Strategies
Step 13: Formulate Improvement Actions
Step 14: Evaluate Proposed Improvement Actions
Step 15: Design Improvements
Step 16: Ensure Acceptability of the Action Plan
Step 17: Implement the Improvement Plan
Step 18: Develop Measures of Effectiveness and Ensure Their Success
Step 19: Evaluate Implementation of Improvement Efforts
Step 20: Take Additional Action
Step 21: Communicate the Results

9 | Step Nine: Identify Which Systems Are Involved—The Root Causes

The probing continues. At this point, the team has a detailed description of the event or "near miss" and a list of proximate causes which describe the patient care processes and other factors that might have caused or contributed to the problem, or could do so in the future. The team has probably also started to collect data on proximate causes. Now the team again asks, "Why did that proximate cause happen? Which systems and processes underlie proximate factors?" The goal of asking questions at this stage is to identify the underlying causes for the proximate causes. For example, in the case of the elderly patient found dead on the floor by her bed, questions might include the following:

- Why was the patient not monitored for an hour to an hour and a half?

- Why was a new graduate nurse assigned to this patient's care? Did the nurse have the assistance of ancillary staff?
- How much orientation had the nurse completed?
- Why was the patient given a sedative?
- Why was the call light not by the patient's hand?

As in all stages of the process, it is critical to keep the team focused on probing for system or common-cause problems, rather than focusing on human errors. Teams often have trouble at this stage of the root cause analysis. The tendency is to stop short after identifying proximate causes and not to probe deeper. The probing must continue until a reason underlying a cause can no longer be identified. This, then, is a root cause.

Underlying causes may involve special-cause variation, common-cause variation, or both. Being special or common is not an inherent characteristic of the cause itself. Rather, it describes the relationship of the cause to a specific process or system. It is possible for the same cause to be a special cause in one process and a common cause in another. A flowchart of the process(es) at this stage may be very helpful.

Tool: Flowchart

For a special cause in a process, teams should search for the common cause in the system of which the process is a part. Keep asking, "Why did the special-cause variation occur?" to identify one or more common-cause variations in the supporting systems that may represent root causes. There should be a review of the processes and subprocesses that compose the system. This examination should include a review of existing policies and procedures by the process owners in comparison with the actual practice. Any variations should be evaluated for the extent of common-cause variation and the presence of special-cause variation. Leaders need to oversee the linkages of processes and subprocesses within the system.

> **Tip: Clarify All Issues**
> It is critical at this point for the team to clearly define the issues regarding the sentinel event or "near miss" and to be sure that team members share a common understanding of the issues. No matter how obvious the issues may seem, individual team members may not understand them in the same way.
>
> For example, a staff member may not consider identification of the surgical site by *all* operating room team members to be worth the time involved. Or, if a patient suffers a burn during surgery, surgical team members may not agree about whether the burn could have been affected by the proximity of the oxygen cannula to the cautery or how the cannula was handled during the cauterizing procedure.

For example, a special cause is created when one group of surgeons and their assistants do not follow hospital procedures for hand hygiene and this results in a sentinel event. This special cause might be part of a common-cause variation in a larger system: The hospital experiences high rates of postoperative infections resulting from insufficient education in sterile techniques and hand washing. Use Worksheet 5-1, page 103, to organize the team's probe for underlying causes.

Sentinel events and "near misses" can be very complex and involve multiple causes. Understanding causes is essential if the organization is to create lasting improvements. Certain tools can be particularly helpful in systematically looking at an event to determine its causes. Such tools include flowcharts, cause-and-effect diagrams, barrier analysis, failure mode and effects analysis (FMEA), and fault tree analysis. The tools are designed to help root cause analysis team members understand processes and factors that contribute to both good and problematic performance. Groups can also use the tools to study a process. None of the tools requires a statistical background. They may be used singly or in combination to show the relationship between processes and factors, reach conclusions, and systematically analyze causes.

 Tools: *Flowchart, cause-and-effect diagram, barrier analysis, FMEA, fault tree analysis*

Cause-and-effect diagrams or fishbone diagrams are particularly helpful in categorizing and visualizing multiple system or process problems that have contributed to a sentinel event or near miss. The standard categories coming off the main "spine" include people, procedures, equipment or materials, environment, and policies. Such categories as communication, education, leadership, and culture may also be appropriate. Subcauses branch off each major category.

Listing and categorizing the possible causal factors represent a logical starting point in the team's effort to determine the systems involved with the event or near miss. Common or root causes of a sentinel event in a health care organization can be categorized according to the important organization functions or processes performed by the organization. These include processes for the following:
- Human resources
- Information management
- Environmental management
- Leadership—embracing corporate culture, encouragement of communication, and clear communication of priorities

In addition, factors beyond an organization's control should be considered a separate category. Organizations must exercise caution in assigning factors to this category, however. Although a causative factor may be beyond an organization's control, the *protection* of patients from the effects of the uncontrollable factor is within the organization's control, in most cases, and should be addressed as a risk reduction strategy.

Concrete questions about each function mentioned previously can help team members reach the essence of the problem—the systems that lie behind or underneath problematic processes. At this stage, questions can be worded in the following form: "To what degree does . . .?" Follow-up questions for each could be "Can this be improved, and if so, how?" and "What are the pros and cons of expending the necessary resources to improve this?" *See* Sidebar 5-1, pages 96-97, for a full itemization of possible questions.

Other questions may emerge in the course of an analysis. All questions should be fully considered. One team investigating a patient suicide found that systems involving human resources, information management, environmental management, and leadership issues were root causes of the sentinel event:
- In the human resources area, age-specific staff competence had not been assessed adequately, and staff needed additional training in management of suicidal patients.
- In the information management area, information about the patient's past admission was not available. Communication delays resulted in failure to implement appropriate preventive actions.
- In the environmental management area, the team found that access to the appropriate unit for the patient was denied.

Checklist 5-1, pages 98-99, might provide a handy way to ensure that the team has considered selected system-based issues. Readers might wish to refer to Figure 1-2, page 16, in Chapter 1 for a list of the systems or processes that should be considered and investigated for each type of sentinel event.

Another proposed classification system for causal factors is geared more to a manufacturing environment. However, it may be helpful to review this and other classification systems to ensure that the team has identified all possible causal factors. This causal factor category list follows[1]:

Sidebar 5-1. Root Cause Analysis Questions

The following questions may be used to probe for systems problems that underlie problematic processes.

Questions concerning human resource issues may include the following:

- To what degree are staff members properly qualified and currently competent for their responsibilities? Can these be improved, and if so, how? What are the pros and cons of expending the necessary resources to improve these?
- How does actual staffing compare with ideal levels? Can this be improved, and if so, how? What are the pros and cons of expending the necessary resources to improve this?
- What are the plans for dealing with contingencies that tend to reduce effective staffing levels? Can this be improved and, if so, how? What are the pros and cons of expending the necessary resources to improve this?
- To what degree is staff performance in the operant processes addressed? Can this be improved and, if so, how? What are the pros and cons of expending the necessary resources to improve this?
- How can orientation and in-service training be improved? What are the pros and cons of expending the necessary resources to improve this?

Questions concerning information management issues may include the following:

- To what degree is all necessary information available when needed? What are the barriers to information availability and access? To what degree is the information accurate and complete? To what degree is the information unambiguous? Can these factors be improved and, if so, how? What are the pros and cons of expending the necessary resources to improve in this area?
- To what degree is the communication of information among participants adequate? Can this be improved and, if so, how? What are the pros and cons of expending the necessary resources to improve this?

Questions concerning environmental management issues may include the following:

- To what degree is the physical environment appropriate for the processes being carried out? Can this be improved and, if so, how? What are the pros and cons of expending the necessary resources to improve this?
- To what degree are systems in place to identify environmental risks? Can this be improved and, if so, how? What are the pros and cons of expending the necessary resources to improve this?
- What emergency and failure-mode responses have been planned and tested? Can this be improved and, if so, how? What are the pros and cons of expending the necessary resources to improve this?

> **Sidebar 5-1. Root Cause Analysis Questions,** *continued*
>
> **Questions concerning leadership issues may include the following:**
>
> - To what degree is the culture conducive to risk identification and reduction? Can this be improved and, if so, how? What are the pros and cons of expending the necessary resources to improve this?
> - What are the barriers to communication of potential risk factors? Can this be improved and, if so, how? What are the pros and cons of expending the necessary resources to improve this?
> - To what degree is the prevention of adverse outcomes communicated as a high priority? How is this communicated? Can this be improved and, if so, how? What are the pros and cons of expending the necessary resources to improve this?
>
> **Questions concerning uncontrollable factors may include the following:**
>
> - What can be done to protect against the effects of uncontrollable factors? What are the pros and cons of expending the necessary resources to improve this area?

Human Factors

- Verbal communication: The spoken presentation or exchange of information
- Written procedures and documents: The written presentation or exchange of information
- Man-machine interface: The design of equipment used to communicate information from the plan to a person
- Environmental conditions: The physical conditions of a work area
- Work schedule: Factors that contribute to the ability of a worker to perform his or her assigned task in an effective manner
- Work practices: Methods workers use to ensure safe and timely completion of tasks
- Work organization/planning: The work-related tasks including planning, identifying the scope of, assigning responsible individuals to, and scheduling the task to be performed
- Supervisory methods: Techniques used to directly control work-related tasks; in particular, a method used to direct workers in the accomplishment of tasks
- Training/qualification: How a training program is developed and the process of presenting information on how a task is to be performed prior to accomplishing the task
- Change management: The process whereby the hardware or software associated with a particular operation, technique, or system is modified
- Resource management: The process whereby manpower and material are allocated for a particular task/objective
- Managerial methods: An administrative technique used to control or direct work-related plan activities, which includes the process whereby manpower and material are allocated for a particular task objective

Equipment Factors

- Design configuration and analysis: The design layout of a system or subsystem needed to support plan operation and maintenance
- Equipment condition: The failure mechanism of the equipment is the physical cause of the failure
- Environmental conditions: The physical conditions of the equipment area
- Equipment specification, manufacture, and construction: The process that includes the manufacture and installation of equipment in a plant
- Maintenance/testing: The process of maintaining components/systems in optimum conditions
- Plant/system operation: The actual performance of the equipment or component when performing its intended function

Checklist 5-1. Problematic Systems or Processes

Use this checklist to identify and rank problematic systems or processes. Use a 1 to indicate a problem that is a primary factor and a 2 to indicate a problem that is a contributing factor.

Human Resources Issues
___ Qualifications of staff
   ___ Defined
   ___ Verified
   ___ Reviewed and updated on a regular basis
___ Qualifications of physicians
   ___ Defined
   ___ Verified
   ___ Reviewed and updated on a regular basis
___ Qualifications of agency staff
   ___ Defined
   ___ Verified
   ___ Reviewed and updated on a regular basis
___ Training of staff
   ___ Adequacy of training program content
   ___ Receipt of necessary training
   ___ Competence/proficiency testing following training
___ Training of physicians
   ___ Adequacy of training program content
   ___ Receipt of necessary training
   ___ Competence/proficiency testing following training
___ Training of agency staff
   ___ Adequacy of training program content
   ___ Receipt of necessary training
   ___ Competence/proficiency testing following training
___ Competence of staff
   ___ Initially verified
   ___ Reviewed and verified on a regular basis
___ Competence of physicians
   ___ Initially verified
   ___ Reviewed and verified on a regular basis
___ Competence of agency staff
   ___ Initially verified
   ___ Reviewed and verified on a regular basis
___ Supervision of staff
   ___ Adequate for new employees
   ___ Adequate for high-risk activities
___ Current staffing levels
   ___ Based on a reasonable patient acuity measure
   ___ Based on reasonable work loads
___ Current scheduling practices
   ___ Overtime expectations
   ___ Time for work activities
   ___ Time between shifts for shift changes

Information Management Issues
___ Availability of information
___ Accuracy of information
___ Thoroughness of information
___ Clarity of information
___ Communication of information between relevant individuals/participants

Environmental Management Issues
___ Physical environment
   ___ Appropriateness to processes being carried out
   ___ Lighting
   ___ Temperature control
   ___ Noise control
   ___ Size/design of space

Checklist 5-1. Problematic Systems or Processes, *continued*

___ Exposure to infection risks
___ Cleanliness
___ Systems to identify environmental risks
  ___ Quality control activities
  ___ Adequacy of procedures and techniques
  ___ Inspections
  ___ Planned, tested, and implemented emergency and failure-mode responses

Leadership and Communication Issues
___ Culture conducive to risk reduction
___ Corrective actions identified and implemented
___ Risk reduction initiatives receive priority attention
___ Barriers to communication of risks and errors
___ Communication
  ___ Present, as appropriate
  ___ Appropriate method
  ___ Understood
  ___ Timely
  ___ Adequate
___ Managerial controls and policies
  ___ Appropriate controls and policies in place
  ___ Policies enforced
  ___ Communication regarding policy changes

External Factor
- External: Human or nonhuman influence outside the usual control of the company

Step Ten: Prune the List of Root Causes

10 The team's list of causal factors may be lengthy. Regardless of its length or the technique used, the team should analyze each cause or factor. This involves using reasoning skills based on logic. Asking two questions helps clarify whether each cause or problem listed is actually a true root cause:

1. If we fix this problem, will the problem recur in the future?
2. If this problem is a root cause, how does it explain what happened or what could have happened?

One method is using three criteria to determine whether each cause is a root cause or a contributing (or proximate) cause:[2]

1. The problem would not have occurred had the cause not been present.
2. The problem will not recur due to the same causal factor if the cause is corrected or eliminated.
3. Correction or elimination of the cause will prevent recurrence of similar conditions.

If these statements are converted to positive questions and a "no" answer is obtained, the problem is a root cause. If a "yes" answer is obtained, the problem is a contributing/proximate cause. Again, it may be helpful to develop a checklist with these questions built in.

A sample checklist with the questions appears as Checklist 5-2, page 100.

Step Eleven: Confirm Root Causes and Consider Their Interrelationships

11 It is highly likely that the team will identify more than one root cause for a sentinel event or "near miss." Even in those very rare instances when a sentinel event results from the *intentional* act of an individual, more than one root cause is likely (for example, personnel screening, communication, and so forth). Sentinel events in industry tend to have two to four root causes, and these root causes tend to be interrelated. To date, the Joint Commission's Sentinel Event Database indicates four to six root causes identified by participating organizations for each sentinel event.

Checklist 5-2. Differentiating Root Causes and Contributing Causes

To differentiate root causes from contributing causes, ask the following questions of each of the causes on the team's list. If the answer is "no" to each of the three questions, the cause is a root cause. If the answer is "yes" to any one of the three questions, the cause is a contributing cause.

Cause #1 _____

Would the problem have occurred if Cause #1 had not been present?
☐ No = root cause   ☐ Yes = contributing cause

Will the problem recur due to the same causal factor if Cause #1 is corrected or eliminated?
☐ No = root cause   ☐ Yes = contributing cause

Will correction or elimination of Cause #1 lead to similar events?
☐ No = root cause   ☐ Yes = contributing cause

Cause #2 _____

Would the problem have occurred if Cause #2 had not been present?
☐ No = root cause   ☐ Yes = contributing cause

Will the problem recur due to the same causal factor if Cause #2 is corrected or eliminated?
☐ No = root cause   ☐ Yes = contributing cause

Will correction or elimination of Cause #2 lead to similar events?
☐ No = root cause   ☐ Yes = contributing cause

Cause #3 _____

Would the problem have occurred if Cause #3 had not been present?
☐ No = root cause   ☐ Yes = contributing cause

Will the problem recur due to the same causal factor if Cause #3 is corrected or eliminated?
☐ No = root cause   ☐ Yes = contributing cause

Will correction or elimination of Cause #3 lead to similar events?
☐ No = root cause   ☐ Yes = contributing cause

For example, organizations that experienced a sentinel event related to **restraint use** reviewed by the Joint Commission identified the following root causes[3].
- Insufficient staff orientation or training
- Patient assessment, such as incomplete medical assessment or incomplete examination of the individual (for example, failure to identify contraband, such as matches)
- Communication issues
- Inadequate care planning, such as alternatives not fully considered, restraints used as punishment, and inappropriate room or unit assignment
- Staff-related factors such as issues with competency review or credentialing or insufficient staffing levels
- Unsafe equipment or equipment use such as use of split side rails without side rail protectors, use of a high-neck vest, incorrect application of a restraining device, or a monitor or an alarm not working or not being used when appropriate

Organizations that experienced **suicides** in a 24-hour care setting reviewed by the Joint Commission identified the following root causes:[4]
- The environment of care, such as the presence of nonbreakaway bars, rods, or safety rails; lack of testing of breakaway hardware; and inadequate security
- Patient assessment methods, such as incomplete suicide risk assessment at intake, absent or incomplete reassessment, and incomplete examination of patients (for example, failure to identify contraband)
- Staff-related factors, such as insufficient orientation or training, incomplete competency review or credentialing, and inadequate staffing levels
- Communication issues
- Information-related factors, such as incomplete communication among caregivers and information being unavailable when needed

Organizations that experienced **infant abductions** reviewed by the Joint Commission identified the following root causes[5].

- Physical environmental factors such as no line of sight to entry points as well as unmonitored elevator or stairwell access to postpartum and nursery areas
- Security equipment factors such as security equipment not being available, operational, or used as intended
- Staff-related factors such as insufficient orientation/training, competency/credentialing issues, and insufficient staffing levels
- Communication issues

Root causes of **medication errors**[6] include communication issues, storage/access issues, insufficient orientation/training, competency/credentialing issues, insufficient staffing levels, and lack of procedural compliance.

Root causes of **wrong-site surgery**[7] include miscommunication by operating room teams, insufficient orientation and training of staff, lack of procedural compliance, lack of available information, distraction, and leadership issues.

Root causes of death or serious injury due to **treatment delays**[8] include inadequate communication among caregivers, insufficient patient assessment, continuum of care issues, insufficient staff orientation and training, inadequate availability of information, and insufficient competency/credentialing processes.

Root causes of sentinel events related to **patient falls**[9] include insufficient staff orientation and training, inadequate caregiver communication, inadequate assessment and reassessment, an unsafe environment of care, and inadequate care planning and provision. Although this information may provide insight into areas to explore, organizations should not rely exclusively on these lists, but should uncover their own unique root causes.

The identification of *all* root causes is essential to preventing a failure or "near miss." Why? Because the interaction of the root causes is likely to be at the root of the problem. If an organization eliminates only one root cause, it has reduced the likelihood of that one very specific adverse outcome occurring again. But if the organization misses the other five root causes, it is possible that those root causes could interact in another way to cause a different but equally adverse outcome. The root causes collectively represent, in effect, latent conditions that could occur. *Latent conditions* are in effect, accidents or sentinel events waiting to happen. The combination of root causes sets the stage for sentinel events. Effective identification of *all* root causes and an understanding of their interaction can aid organizations in changing processes to eliminate a whole family of risks, not just a single risk. Elimination of only one of the root causes mentioned previously does not eliminate the risk inherent in the processes addressing restraint use, the prevention of suicide in a 24-hour care setting, infant abduction, or other sentinel events.

For example, with the restraint use case, to eliminate the root cause of unsafe equipment use, staff can be trained in selecting safe equipment and using it safely. However, what happens six months later when an individual staff member has forgotten how to use a four-point restraint properly? Does the organization have an effective plan for assessing the continued competence of the staff member to use restraint safely and to provide follow-up training when necessary? What happens if restraint is required when agency staff are on duty? Are they trained and competent to use restraint safely? After a patient is placed in restraint, does the staff member know how to consistently observe the patient in restraint according to organization policies and procedures (for example, to *detect* the result of a mistake in the restraint application process or an equipment failure)? Each of the root causes is interrelated to others. Elimination of a single root cause does not eliminate the latent conditions waiting to happen.

If a team identifies more than six root causes, a number of the causes may be defined too specifically. In this case, the team may wish to review whether one or more of the root causes could logically be combined with another to reflect more basic, system-oriented causes. The team should verify each of the remaining root causes. This involves cross-checking for accuracy and consistency all facts, tools, and techniques used to analyze information. Any inconsistencies and discrepancies should be resolved.

How does an organization know whether and when it has identified *all* true root causes of a sentinel event? Try using a checklist to determine whether the team has identified all root causes.

A team should report its root cause findings to the leaders of its organization. Leaders must be informed, as should the individuals likely to be impacted by changes emerging from the findings, during the next stage of the root cause analysis. See Chapter 6 for more information on communicating the results of the team's efforts.

References

1. Ammerman M.: *The Root Cause Analysis Handbook: A Simplified Approach to Identifying, Correcting, and Reporting Workplace Errors.* New York: Quality Resources, 1998, pp. 66–67.
2. Ammerman, pp. 68–69.
3. Joint Commission: Root Causes of Restraint Deaths (1995–2004). http://www.jcaho.org/accredited+organizations/ambulatory +care/sentinel+events/rc+restraint+deaths.htm.
4. Joint Commission: Root Causes of Inpatient Suicides (1995–2004). http://www.jcaho.org/accredited+organizations/ambulatory +care/sentinel+events/rc+inpatient+suicides.htm.
5. Joint Commission: Root Causes of Infant Abductions (1995–2004). http://www.jcaho.org/accredited+organizations/ambulatory +care/sentinel+events/rc+infant+abductions.htm.
6. Joint Commission: Root Causes of Medication Errors (1995–2004). http://www.jcaho.org/accredited+organizations/ambulatory +care/sentinel+events/rc+of+medication+errors.htm.
7. Joint Commission: Root Causes of Wrong-Site Surgery (1995–2004). http://www.jcaho.org/accredited+organizations/ambulatory +care/sentinel+events/rc+wrong+site+surgery.htm.
8. Joint Commission: Root Causes of Delays in Treatment (1995–2004). http://www.jcaho.org/accredited+organizations/ambulatory +care/sentinel+events/rc+of+delay+in+treatment.htm.
9. Joint Commission: Root Causes of Patient Falls (1995–2004). http://www.jcaho.org/accredited+organizations/ambulatory+care/ sentinel+events/rc+of+patient+falls.htm.

Worksheet 5-1. Probing for Underlying Causes

The team might find it helpful to use a worksheet when probing for the underlying causes of proximate causes. For example, with the fire-related death of a restrained patient, the worksheet could be organized (and begun) as follows:

Proximate Causes

1. Missed observation

2. Patient possessed contraband matches

3. _____

4. _____

5. _____

Underlying Causes

Staff training and orientation

Staffing model

Patient observation procedures

Suicide risk assessment procedure

_____

_____

_____

Chapter 6
Designing and Implementing an Action Plan for Improvement

In previous chapters, identifying the proximate and root causes of a sentinel event or "near miss" was discussed. The final and perhaps most important stage of the root cause analysis process involves identifying risk reduction strategies; setting priorities and objectives for improvement in areas identified as at the root of the problem; and developing, implementing, and measuring the effectiveness of improvement efforts. This chapter covers these topics in workbook format. Figure 1-3, pages 20-23, from Chapter 1 provides the framework for this step of the analysis.

Step 1: Organize a Team
Step 2: Define the Problem
Step 3: Study the Problem
Step 4: Determine What Happened
Step 5: Identify Contributing Process Factors
Step 6: Identify Other Contributing Factors
Step 7: Measure—Collect and Assess Data on Proximate and Underlying Causes
Step 8: Design and Implement Interim Changes
Step 9: Identify Which Systems Are Involved—The Root Causes
Step 10: Prune the List of Root Causes
Step 11: Confirm Root Causes and Consider Their Interrelationships
Step 12: Explore and Identify Risk Reduction Strategies
Step 13: Formulate Improvement Actions
Step 14: Evaluate Proposed Improvement Actions
Step 15: Design Improvements
Step 16: Ensure Acceptability of the Action Plan
Step 17: Implement the Improvement Plan
Step 18: Develop Measures of Effectiveness and Ensure Their Success
Step 19: Evaluate Implementation of Improvement Efforts
Step 20: Take Additional Action
Step 21: Communicate the Results

12 Step Twelve: Explore and Identify Risk Reduction Strategies

The team asks, "So what are we going to do with the problematic systems now that we have identified them?" When the team has a solid hypothesis about one or more root causes, the next step is to explore and identify risk reduction strategies to help ensure that faulty systems are improved for the future.

The team might start by exploring relevant literature on risk reduction and error-prevention strategies. Much has been written about the engineering approach to failure prevention and how it differs from the medical approach. Some of the literature's key points are described here.

The pervasive view of errors in the engineering field is that humans err frequently and that the cause of an error is often beyond the individual's control. In designing systems and processes, engineers begin with the premise that anything can and will go wrong. Their role is a proactive one—to design accordingly. Because engineering-based industries do not expect individuals to perform flawlessly, they try to design systems that make it difficult for individuals to make mistakes. By compensating for less-than-perfect human performance, engineering systems achieve a high degree of reliability through backup systems and designed redundancy. A failure rate even as low as 1% is not tolerated. The emphasis is on systems rather than individuals.

In contrast, the still-pervasive view in the health care field is that errors are the result of individual human failure and that humans generally perform flawlessly. Hence, processes in health care organizations tend to be designed based on the premise that nothing will go wrong. Education and training, more extensive in health care than in most other fields, focus on teaching professionals to do the right thing. The assumption is that properly educated and trained health care professionals will not make mistakes. Those that do are retrained, punished, or sanctioned. The immediate causes of errors are identified and corrected, but not planned or designed for. Root causes are rarely identified.

Lucian L. Leape, MD, has done much work comparing risk reduction approaches in various industries to those in the health care industry. He suggests four safety design characteristics from the aviation industry that could, with some modification, prove useful in improving safety in the health care industry[1]:

- Built-in multiple buffers, automation, and redundancy. Instrumentation in airplane cockpits includes multiple and purposely redundant monitoring instruments. The design systems assume that errors and failures are inevitable and should be absorbed.
- Standardized procedures. Protocols that must be followed exist for operating and maintaining airplanes.
- A highly developed and rigidly enforced training, examination, and certification process. Pilots take proficiency exams every six months.
- Institutionalized safety. The airline industry reports directly to two agencies that regulate all aspects of flying, prescribe safety procedures, and investigate all accidents. A confidential safety reporting system established by the Federal Aviation Administration enables pilots, controllers, or others to report dangerous situations, including errors they have made, to a third party without penalty. This program greatly increases error reporting in aviation, resulting in enhanced communication and prompt problem solving.

Planning risk reduction strategies should consider three levels of design to reduce the risk of harm to patients: (1) design the process to minimize the risk of a failure; (2) design the process to minimize the risk that a failure will reach the patient; (3) design the process to mitigate the effects of a failure that reaches the patient. An example of a consideration for the first level of design is ensuring a positive interlock between tubes in a ventilator airflow circuit that might prevent a failure such as an inadvertent disconnection of the tubes. On the second level of design, an example of a consideration is ensuring that an airway pressure alarm that can detect a pressure drop due to a tubing disconnection and alert staff before a patient is harmed is in place. An example of a consideration for the third level of design is the ready availability of resuscitation equipment that can mitigate the effect of oxygen deprivation due to a prolonged tubing disconnection. It is also critical that error-prevention strategies used in the health care industry include standardizing tasks and processes to minimize reliance on weak aspects of cognition, testing of professional performance, and institutionalizing safety through "near miss" and nonpunitive reporting. For example, clinical practice guidelines and organization policies and protocols designed to reduce inappropriate variation in the care provided by practitioners can help reduce the likelihood of failures.

Risk reduction strategies must emphasize a systems rather than an individual human approach. A system can be thought of as any collection of components and the relationships between them, whether the components are human or not, when the components have been brought together for a well-defined goal or purpose.[2] As Leape writes, "Creating a safe process, whether it be flying an airplane, running a hospital, or performing cardiac surgery, requires attention to methods of error reduction at each stage of system development: design, construction, maintenance, allocation of resources, training, and development of operational procedures."[3] If errors are made, if deficiencies are discovered, individuals at each stage must revisit previous decisions and redesign or reorganize the process.

Designing for safety means making it difficult for humans to err. However, those designing systems must recognize that failures occur and that recovery or correction should be built into the system. If this is not possible, failures must be capable of being detected promptly so that individuals have time to take corrective actions. For example, as required by the Universal Protocol for Preventing Wrong Site, Wrong Procedure, Wrong Person Surgery™, a preoperative verification process such as a checklist must be used to confirm that appropriate documents (such as medical records and imaging studies) are available. The Universal Protocol also states that a process must be implemented to mark the surgical site and the patient must be involved in the marking process. In addition, a check by the circulating nurse and checks conducted directly with the patient and family facilitate the detection of potential wrong-site surgical errors.

Risk points—specific points in a process that are susceptible to failure or system breakdown—must be eliminated through design or redesign efforts (*see* Chapter 3. Built-in buffers and redundancy, task and process simplification and standardization, and training are all appropriate design mechanisms to reduce the likelihood of failure at risk points and elsewhere.

For example, prior to the administration of medications, multiple and redundant checks, such as asking the patient his or her name and checking the patient's armband can help confirm that a drug is given to the right patient. *See* Sidebar 6-1, page 108, for risk points for medication errors and risk reduction strategies to prevent such failures.

Risk points and risk reduction strategies for wrong-site surgery, restraint-related deaths, suicide, and infant abductions or release to wrong families follow. Readers should note that a number of these strategies are not specific Joint Commission requirements, but are presented for consideration by all health care organizations.

Risk points for **wrong-site surgery** include the following:
- Communication before reaching operating suite
- Communication in operating suite
- Hierarchical issues of communication
- Communication with patient/family
- Information availability
- Multiple surgery sites
- Conflicting chart information
- Confused patient
- X-ray quality/accuracy

Risk reduction strategies to reduce the likelihood of failures associated with *preoperative procedures* include the following:
- Mark operative site.
- Require surgeon to obtain informed consent.
- Require preoperative verification by surgeon, anesthesiologist/anesthetist, and patient or family.
- Personally review X-rays.
- Revise equipment setup procedures.

To reduce the likelihood of failures in the *operating suite*, do the following:
- Verify before prep and drape.
- Make sure site marking is visible after draping.
- Obtain verbal verification with a timeout.
- Confirm level of spinal surgery with intraoperative fluoroscopy.

Sidebar 6-1. Medication Errors: Risk Points and Risk Reduction Strategies

Risk points or common causes:
- Inadequate training/education
- Competence (lapses in performance, failure to comply with policies and procedures)
- Supervision
- Staffing (excessive workload, incorrect mix)
- Communication failures
- Distraction due to environmental issues
- Information availability
- Medication storage/access
- Labeling
- Nomenclature
- Dosage calculation
- Equipment failure
- Abbreviations
- Handwriting

Risk reduction strategies:
To reduce the likelihood of failures associated with *prescribing* errors:
- Implement a system of computerized order entry by physicians (to decrease the likelihood of dosage error, prompt for allergies, and provide information on drug-drug and drug-food interactions).
- Redefine the role of pharmacists to enable them to perform daily rounds with physicians, work with registered nurses, and serve as on-site resources.

To reduce the likelihood of failures associated with *dispensing*:
- Do not rely on color-coding.
- Remove look-alikes/sound-alikes.
- Bar code if possible.
- Avoid lethal medications in bolus form.
- Use premixed solutions, when possible.
- Minimize supplier/product changes.
- Use auxiliary labels ("such as, for IM [intramuscular] only").
- Support questioning of unclear orders.
- Eliminate guessing.

To reduce the likelihood of failures associated with *access* to medications:
- Remove high-risk medications from care units.
- Label high-risk medications as such.
- Establish and implement policies and procedures for use of off-hours pharmacy.

To reduce the likelihood of failures associated with *medication delivery*:
- Be sure that equipment defaults to the least harmful mode.
- Use automated pharmacy units as a tool for improving the process, not an inherent solution.
- Recognize that polypharmacy equals higher risk.

To reduce the likelihood of failures associated with *human resources and competence factors*:
- Address education and training issues (orientation, competence assessment, and training with new medications and devices).
- Support professional ethics and judgment.
- Implement systems involving double checks.
- Make safe staffing choices.
- Tackle illegible handwriting.
- Discourage use of acronyms and abbreviations.
- Control availability of high-risk drugs.
- Address environmental issues. (Tackle distraction and its impact.)
- Standardize medication times.
- Use patients as safety partners.

Risk points for **restraint use** include the following:
- Restraining patients with high-risk factors, including those who smoke, who have deformities that preclude proper fit of restraints, who have potentially compromised protective reflexes (such as those under conscious sedation or those profoundly intoxicated)
- Restraining patients in supine position, increasing risk of aspiration
- Restraining patients in prone position, increasing risk of suffocation
- Restraining patients in room not under continuous observation

Risk reduction strategies include the following:
- Do not restrain a patient in bed with unprotected, split side rails.
- Never use a towel, bag, or cover over a patient's face.
- Ensure that all smoking materials are removed from a patient's access.
- Continuously observe any patient who is restrained.
- Educate staff on appropriate use and alternative measures.
- Revise the staffing model.
- Ensure staff competence and training.
- Use less-restrictive measures, and increase and standardize choices.
- Revise policy and procedures regarding assessment.

Strategies to reduce the risk of **suicide** in a staffed round-the-clock care setting include the following:
- Revise assessment/reassessment procedures and assure adherence.
- Update the staffing model.
- Educate staff on suicide risk factors.
- Update policies on patient observation.
- Monitor consistency of implementation.
- Revise information transfer procedures.
- Revisit contraband policies.
- Identify and remove nonbreakaway hardware.
- Weight test all breakaway hardware.
- Redesign or retrofit security measures.
- Educate family and friends on suicide risk factors.
- Consider patients in all areas.
- Ensure that staff members ask about suicidal thoughts every shift.
- Be cautious at times of shift change (admission, discharge, passes).
- Avoid reliance on pacts.
- Be suspicious if symptoms lighten suddenly.
- Involve all staff in solutions.

Strategies to reduce the risk of **infant abductions** include the following:
- Develop and implement a proactive infant abduction prevention plan.
- Include information on visitor/provider identification as well as identification of potential abductors/abduction situations during staff orientation and in-service curriculum programs.
- Enhance parent education concerning abduction risks and parent responsibility for reducing risk, and then assess the parents' level of understanding.
- Attach secure identically numbered bands to the baby (wrist and ankle bands), mother, and father or significant other immediately after birth.
- Footprint the baby, take a color photograph of the baby, and record the baby's physical examination within two hours of birth.
- Require staff to wear up-to-date, conspicuous, color photograph identification badges.
- Discontinue publication of birth notices in local newspapers.
- Consider options for controlling access to the nursery/postpartum unit such as swipe-card locks, keypad locks, entry point alarms, or video surveillance. (Any locking systems must comply with fire codes.)
- Consider implementing an infant security tag or abduction alarm system.

Systems engineering literature includes numerous other design concepts that could be useful tools to prevent failures and sentinel events in health care organizations. *Redundancy* is one such concept familiar to the aerospace and nuclear power industries,

Checklist 6-1. Identifying Risk Reduction Strategies

To reduce the likelihood of failures, the medical and engineering literature offers the following tips:
- ☐ Use an engineering approach to failure prevention.
- ☐ Start with the premise that anything can and will go wrong.
- ☐ Design systems that make the safest thing to do the easiest thing to do.
- ☐ Design systems that make it difficult for individuals to err.
- ☐ Build in as much redundancy as possible.
- ☐ Use fail-safe design whenever possible.
- ☐ Simplify and standardize procedures.
- ☐ Automate procedures.
- ☐ Ensure rigidly enforced training and competence assessment processes.
- ☐ Ensure nonpunitive reporting of "near misses."
- ☐ Eliminate risk points.

---

device. If the satellite or missile misses its target within a set time, the destruct system blows the satellite or missile apart to halt its flight and limit any damage it might cause by falling to the ground. Checklist 6-1, left, provides the key risk reduction strategies suggested in the medical and engineering literature.

Tool: *Failure mode and effects analysis (FMEA)*

Failure mode and effects analysis (FMEA) can be used to identify risk reduction opportunities. Also known in the literature as failure mode, effects, and criticality analysis (FMECA), FMEA offers a systematic way of examining a design prospectively for possible ways in which failure can occur. Potential failures are identified in terms of failure modes or symptoms, as opposed to causes. For each failure mode, the effect on the total system or process is studied. Actions (planned or already taken) can be reviewed for their potential to minimize the probability of failure or the effects of failure. FMEA's goal is to prevent poor results, which in health care means harm to patients. Its greatest strength lies in its capability to focus users on the process of redesigning potentially problematic processes to prevent the occurrence of failures.

Although the technique has been used very effectively in the engineering world since the 1960s, its use in the health care world began as late as the 1990s. FMEA is now gaining broader acceptance in health care as a tool for prospective analysis due to the efforts of the Joint Commission, VA National Center for Patient Safety, and the Institute for Safe Medication Practices, among others. In 2002, the Joint Commission published the first book on FMEA's application in health care[4] (now in its second edition) which is intended as a companion publication to this publication. The eight steps involved in an FMEA approach, as outlined by the Joint Commission, appear in Chapter 7, page 159.

where systems have backups and even the backups normally have backups. System reliability can be increased by introducing redundancy into system design. However, the cost of designing in redundancy is an issue in most health care environments. The engineering literature also describes the benefits of simplification, standardization, and loose coupling to reduce the possibility of systems-related problems.

Fail-safe design is also a concept familiar to high-reliability industries, including aerospace and nuclear engineering. The design may be fail-passive, fail-operational, or fail-active. For example, a circuit breaker is a fail-passive device that opens when a dangerous situation occurs, thereby making an electrical system safe. A destruct system on a satellite or an air-to-air missile is an example of a fail-active

FMEA is described here because root cause analysis teams may also wish to use FMEA to proactively identify risk reduction opportunities during their root cause analysis of a sentinel event or near miss or to carry out a proactive risk assessment on a process that is being redesigned in response to the findings of a root cause analysis.

Tool: *Failure mode and effects analysis (FMEA)*

A performance improvement team at a community hospital in Michigan used FMEA for one of the first times in health care to proactively analyze and reduce medication errors associated with potassium chloride (KCl).[5] The focus was on developing strategies to reduce the risk of future fatal errors. The team followed the steps outlined in Table 6-1, right.

The process flow diagram developed by the team for the medication use process from point of initiation through completion appears as Figure 6-1, page 112. The team's outline of what could go wrong and its ranking appears as Table 6-2, page 113. Possible failure-preventing actions appear in Table 6-3, page 114. These are presented as a model to help teams successfully integrate a ranking system.

Step Thirteen: Formulate Improvement Actions

With the list of root causes in hand, the team is now ready to start devising potential solutions to systems-related problems. Known as corrective or improvement actions, these solutions are required to prevent a problem from occurring or recurring due to the same root cause(s) or interaction of root causes. The team may include the same members as during the early stages of the root cause analysis, or new members might be brought on board as required by the recommended improvements.

When formulating improvement actions, think in terms of the everyday work of the organization. Work can be

Table 6-1. Steps in FMEA

1. Set up a process flow diagram.
2. Retrace the process flow diagram, assuming the worst, to figure out what could go wrong along the way.
3. Decide what the effects of failure might be on the remainder of the process.
4. Rank the estimated possibility of occurrence using the following scale: 1=remote possibility; 5=possibility; 10=almost certain.
5. Rank the estimated severity of the overall failure using the following scale: 1=will not cause patient harm; 5=may affect patient adversely; 10=injury or death will occur.
6. Rank the estimated likelihood that failure will be detected before accident takes place: 1=will always be detected; 5=might be detected; 10=detection not possible.
7. Calculate the criticality index (mean of steps 4, 5, and 6).
8. Decide on interventions to lower the criticality index.
9. Take action.
10. Assess.

Source: Cohen M.: Failure mode and effects analysis: Dealing with human error in medicine. *Proceedings of the Physicians Insurance Company of Michigan.* Apr. 1994.

defined in terms of functions or processes. A function is a group of processes with a common goal, and a *process* is a series of linked, goal-directed activities. Improvement actions should be directed primarily at processes. As stated earlier in this book, process improvement holds the greatest opportunity for significant change, whereas changes related to an individual's performance tend to have limited effect. Good people often find themselves carrying out bad processes. System problems identified and resolutions suggested by an interdisciplinary medication incident task force at one organization appear as Table 6-4, page 115.

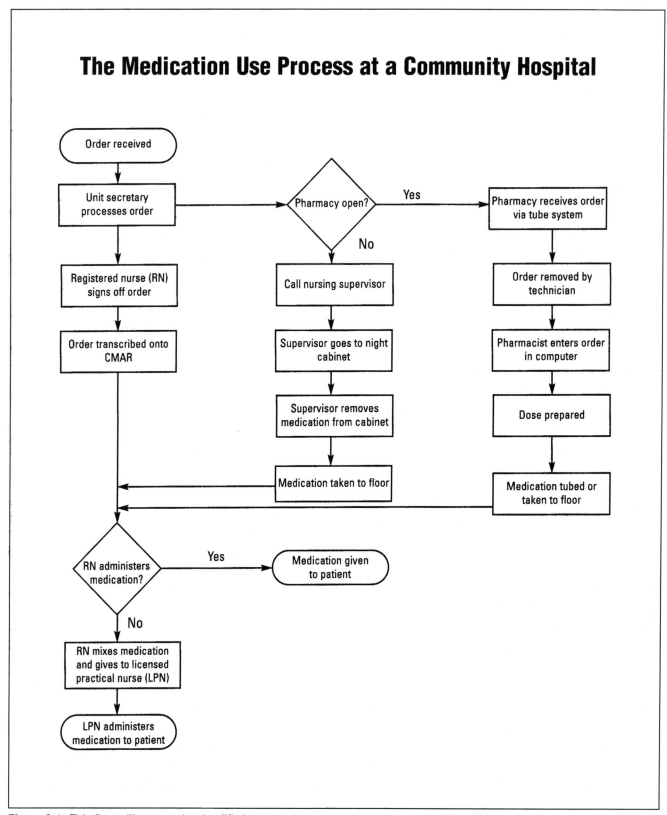

Figure 6-1. This figure illustrates the simplified process flowchart one community hospital created as step one in an FMEA. In step two they went through the flowchart, action by action, to brainstorm what might go wrong. Table 6-2 on page 113 lists the possible failures the hospital brainstormed. CMAR stands for computerized medication administration record.
Source: Fletcher C.E.: Failure and effects analysis. *J Nurs Adm* 27(12):23, 1997.

Table 6-2. Possible Risk Points in the Medication Use Process

Order Received
- Phone order not clarified.
- Verbal order not clarified.
- Written order illegible.
- Dose may be incorrect.
- Incorrect route.
- Order written on wrong chart.
- Order written on right chart, but stamped with wrong name.
- Wrong drug.
- Drug not indicated.
- Language barrier present with verbal phone order.

Unit Secretary Processes Order
- Does not take order out of chart.
- Sends order to department other than pharmacy.
- Misplaces order and does not send it at all.
- Misinterprets and thus processes incorrectly.
- Delays in processing occur.
- Stamps wrong name on order sheet.

Registered Nurse Signs Off Order
- Delays order.
- Does not read order carefully, but processes it anyway.
- Does not take time to read order, but processes it anyway.
- Cosigns order without giving it to secretary; does not go through correct process.
- Cannot read/misreads order.
- Orders added by physician after initial order processed; RN does not see additional orders.
- Unfamiliar with drug: allergy, dose, and/or cross sensitivity.

Order Transcribed onto CMAR
- RN's handwriting unclear.
- Order transcribed onto wrong computerized medical administration record (CMAR).
- Order transcribed incorrectly.
- Order not transcribed in a timely manner.
- Lack of nursing communication to RN or licensed practical nurse (LPN) giving medication.
- Forgetting/failure to transcribe.

RN Mixes Medication
- Miscalculated dose.
- Miscalculated measurement of volume.
- Selects wrong drug.
- Prepares wrong drug brought by supervisor (after hours).
- Does not match the order to the chart.
- Labeling errors: drug is not actually added to IV or IV contains drug but no label.
- Lacks knowledge of administration policies and procedures.
- Lacks knowledge regarding IV versus oral dosing guidelines.
- Interrupted during preparation.
- Lacks routine/organization when doing the task.

RN or LPN Administers Medication to Patient
- Wrong patient.
- Incorrect labeling.
- Intravenous accurate control (IVAC) not used.
- No IVAC available.
- Wrong rate of flow set on IVAC.

Source: Fletcher C.E.: Failure and effects analysis. *J Nurs Adm* 27(12):24, 1997.

Table 6-3. Possible Failure-Preventing Actions

Remove Alternatives
- Eliminate dangerous items and procedures.
- Limit use or access.
- Locate items with care.
- Follow protocols and procedures.
- Ascertain certification or privileging.
- Maintain hospital drug formulary control.
- Avoid potential for confirmation bias. (Minimize look-alike containers, names, computer abbreviations, and so forth.)
- Minimize consequence of error.

Improve Detection
- Orientation, education, additional training.
- Protocols and procedures.
- Redundancy.
- Lock-and-key design.
- Hazard warnings and signs, auxiliary labels, medication administration record (MAR) warnings, and so forth.
- Technology (bar code, computer, and so forth).
- Improved detection process.
- Documentation.
- Tactile cues.

Prevent Completion of Actions
- Fail-safe design.
- Lock and key design.
- Technology.

Minimize Consequence of Failure
- Reduce supply (volume, concentration, number of tablets, vials, and so forth).
- Modify defaults.

Source: Cohen M.: Failure mode and effects analysis: Dealing with human error in medicine. *Proceedings of the Physicians Insurance Company of Michigan.* Apr. 1994.

Returning to the sentinel events described in Chapter 3, consider the following examples of how root cause analysis teams could approach the identification of improvement actions.

In the **suicide** example, the team has completed a cause-and-effect diagram indicating multiple system problems, including assessment of suicide risk, environment of care, and emergency procedures. The team might break into smaller subgroups. One group (including the psychiatrist, medical staff leader, and nurse) would address the failed patient assessment process. They might start by reviewing the current standard for assessment of suicide risk and how this standard is communicated in the behavioral health unit. Another group (including the administrator and plant safety representative) might start working on environment of care issues such as nonbreakaway shower heads. Another group (including emergency department physicians and the nursing staff) might work on emergency procedures.

In the **elopement** example, the root cause analysis team has identified multiple system problems including an unsafe environment of care, inadequate assessment and reassessment; and inadequate staff orientation, training, and ongoing competence assessment. One subgroup (including the safety director, a nurse from the unit, and a social worker) might address possible actions to improve the long term care organization's security and safety measures. Another small group (including the medical director, director of nursing, activity staff member, and unit staff nurse) might address opportunities to improve the

Table 6-4. Sample System Problems and Suggested Resolutions

Problem
- Lack of uniform procedures in medication administration from one unit to another.
- Limited pharmacy involvement in the medication incident reporting and tracking process.
- Controlled drugs frequently involved in ordered drug errors.
- Use of unofficial abbreviations for drug names identified as a source of several unordered drug errors.
- Use of Latin abbreviations such as QD, QOD, and OD and abbreviation U for units identified as a source of errors.
- Physician order sheets were not removed from patients' charts; therefore, pharmacy Kardex was not complete and accurate.

Suggested Resolution
- Assess current unit differences in medication administration procedures by developing a survey instrument. Determine methods to standardize procedures to minimize errors.
- Analyze weekly summary of errors, prepared in the Department of Pharmacy, to determine system defects that may be correctable.
- Investigate automated dispensing systems to minimize errors with controlled substances.
- Form a subcommittee of the Pharmacy and Therapeutics Committee to review this issue and recommend appropriate action.
- Organize subcommittee of the Pharmacy and Therapeutics Committee to prepare a recommendation on the use of abbreviations in an effort to meet the National Patient Safety Goal that addresses the use of abbreviations.
- Collect data to identify areas where this is most common; provide corrective measures to focus on these areas.

Source: Bradbury K., et al.: Prevention of medication errors: Developing a continuous-quality improvement approach. *Mt Sinai J Med* 60(5):382, 1993.

---

process used to assess and reassess patients at risk for elopement. Another group (including the medical director, the director of nursing, and the performance improvement coordinator) might address strategies to ensure that staff know elopement risk factors and who is at risk for elopement and are assessed regularly for competence in identifying and caring for at-risk patients.

In the **treatment delay** example, the team has identified system problems that led to the missed diagnosis of metastasized breast cancer. These include communication problems between caregivers, insufficient staff orientation and training, and inadequate information management. Subgroups of the ambulatory care organization's team probe each of these areas for improvement opportunities, looking at such issues as care documentation and the availability of clinical records, the timeliness and thoroughness of initial and regular reassessments, and shift-to-shift communication of information related to patient needs.

In the **medication error** example, the root cause analysis team has identified communication of medication orders and the failure to ensure safe medication storage and access as two key problems, among others. A subgroup (including the information technology staff member, pharmacist, medical director, and home health nurse) might investigate possible strategies to improve the accuracy of orders communicated to local pharmacies. Another subgroup, including the nursing supervisor, pharmacy supplier, home health nurse, and medical director, might investigate strategies to guard against medication theft and ensure proper implementation of the home health agency's medication administration policies and procedures.

For each root cause, the team should work interactively either as a whole or in smaller groups to develop a list of possible improvement actions. Brainstorming can be used to generate additional ideas. The emphasis at this point is on generating as many improvement actions as possible, not on evaluating the ideas or their feasibility. The number of suggested improvement actions may vary based on the nature of the root cause and how it relates to other root causes. To ensure as thorough a list as possible, the team may wish to review the analyses of information used to identify root causes. Remember to encourage any and all ideas without critiquing them. In the hands of a skilled facilitator, even the seemingly wildest idea can lead to an effective improvement action during later stages of analysis. Tools used such as flowcharts or cause-and-effect diagrams can prompt additional solutions. Ask questions of the group, such as the following:
- What might fix this problem?
- What other solutions can we generate?
- What other ideas haven't we thought of?

Tools: Brainstorming, flowchart, cause-and-effect diagram

Wilson and his colleagues suggest using the scientific method to develop a list of potential solutions. He restates the scientific method in terms of steps used in developing solutions:
- Become familiar with all the aspects of the problem and its causes.
- Derive a number of tentative solutions.
- Assemble as much detail as is needed to clearly define what is required to implement these solutions.
- Evaluate the suggested solutions.
- Objectively test and revise the solutions.
- Develop a final list of potential solutions.[6]

These steps may assist the team through the process of both developing and evaluating improvement actions.

14 Step Fourteen: Evaluate Proposed Improvement Actions

When the list of possible improvement actions is as complete as possible, the team is ready to evaluate the alternatives and select those actions to be recommended to leadership.

To begin the evaluation process, the team should rank the ideas based on criteria defined by the team. Gathering appropriate data is critical to this process. A simple six-point scale ranging from a low rank of 0 for the worst alternative to a high rank of 5 for the best alternative can be used at this point. Spath suggests asking the team to rank the solutions in order of workability, reliability, risk, chance for success, management/staff/physician receptivity, cost, capability to fix the problem, and other factors.[7] To rank the proposed solutions, Ammerman suggests using criteria such as compatibility with other organization commitments and possible creation of other adverse effects.[8]

Initially, to prevent group think, it is a good idea to ask each team member to rank the ideas on his or her own. The rankings can then be consolidated into a team ranking. To keep track of suggested improvement actions, complete Worksheet 6-1, page 134. Record the rankings assigned by individual team members and the team as a whole.

FMEA may be a helpful tool at this point in the process. FMEA involves evaluating potential problems (or improvement actions) and prioritizing or ranking these on a proactive basis according to criteria defined by a team (*see* Table 6-1, page 111, and Chapter 7, page 159).

Tool: *Failure mode and effects analysis (FMEA)*

At the very least, every improvement action proposed by the team should be objective and measurable. If it is objective, implementation is easier and those affected by the change are more likely to be receptive. If it is measurable, the team can ensure that improvement actually occurs. *See* Sidebar 6-2, right, for evaluative criteria for improvement actions. Before ranking the actions, ensure that the team reaches a consensus on which criteria are most relevant to the organization. Ranking the proposed ideas according to multiple criteria adds critical dimension to the evaluation.

In evaluating potential improvement actions, the team should consider the impact of the suggested improvement on organization processes, resources, and schedules. Sentinel events or near misses frequently shake up the organization's notions of the resources that should be expended in particular areas. Organizations contemplating a design or redesign effort will certainly weigh the availability of resources against the potential benefits for patients, customers, and the organization.

Asking some key questions helps the team identify the potential barriers to implementation of each improvement action. Relevant questions include the following.

Organization Processes
- How does the proposed action relate to other projects currently underway in the organization? Are there redundancies?
- How does the action affect other areas and processes?
- What process-related changes might be required?
- Can affected areas absorb the changes/additional responsibilities?

Sidebar 6-2. Evaluating Improvement Actions

- Likelihood of success (preventing recurrence or occurrence) within the organization's capabilities
- Compatibility with organization's objectives
- Risk
- Reliability
- Likelihood to engender other adverse effects
- Receptivity by management/staff/physicians
- Barriers to implementation
- Implementation time
- Long-term (versus short-term) solution
- Cost
- Measurability

Resources
- What financial resources will be required to implement the action? (Include both direct and indirect costs—that is, costs associated with the necessary changes to other procedures and processes.) How will these resources be obtained?
- What other resources (staff, time, management) are required for successful implementation? How will these resources be obtained?
- What resources (capital, staff, time, management) are required for continued effectiveness? How will these resources be obtained?

Schedule
- In what time frame can implementation be completed?
- How will implementation of this action affect other schedules? How can this be handled?
- What initial and ongoing training will be required? How will this impact the schedule and how will its impact be handled?

With answers to these questions in hand, the team can better gauge whether the pluses outweigh the minuses.

After completing this questioning process, the team may wish to revisit the ranking exercises described previously. This can help clarify which corrective improvement actions should be selected. To summarize the potential of each proposed action, the team can ask, "What will result from implementing this action?" and "What would result from not implementing this action?" (as shown in Worksheet 6-2, page 135).

At this point, the team should be ready to select a finite number of improvement actions. Each action must do the following:
- Address a root cause
- Offer a long-term solution to the problem
- Have a greater positive than negative impact on other processes, resources, and schedules
- Be objective and measurable
- Have a clearly defined implementation time line
- Be assignable to staff for implementation

The next section describes how the team designs improvements and develops an action plan covering each of these aspects.

Step Fifteen: Design Improvements

The product of the root cause analysis is an action plan that identifies the strategies that the organization intends to implement to reduce the risk of similar events occurring in the future. The team is now ready to start drafting such a plan. The plan should address the five issues of *what*, *how*, *when*, *who*, and *where* involved in implementing and evaluating the effectiveness of proposed improvement actions.

Issue One: What

Designing *what* involves determining the scope of the actions and specific activities that will be recommended. A clear definition of the goals is critical. To understand the potential effects of the improvement activity, the organization must determine which dimension of performance—efficacy, appropriateness, availability, timeliness, effectiveness, continuity, safety, efficiency, and respect and caring—will be affected. Dimensions of performance, which are Joint Commission constructs, not requirements, describe what is measurable about quality. At times, the relationship between two or more dimensions must be considered. Redesign in response to a sentinel event most often focuses on safety, but may affect any or all the other dimensions. What specific activities will be needed to achieve the necessary improvement? Use Worksheet 6-3, page 136, to articulate responses to questions concerning goals, dimensions of performance, and required specific activities.

Issue Two: How

How does the organization expect, want, and need the improved process to perform? The team carrying out the effort should set specific expectations for performance resulting from the design or improvement. Without these expectations, the organization cannot determine the degree of success of the efforts. These expectations can be derived from staff expertise, consumer expectations, experiences of other organizations, recognized standards, and other sources. What sequence of activities and resources will be required to meet these expectations? How and what will the team measure to determine whether the process is actually performing at the level expected?

The organization or group needs specific tools to measure the performance of the newly designed or improved process to determine whether expectations are met. These measures can be taken directly, adapted from other sources, or newly created, as appropriate. It is important for the measures to be as quantitative as possible. This means that the measurement can be represented by a scale or range of values. For example, if improving staff competence in calculating medication doses is cited as a corrective solution, the measure should evaluate competence before and after each training or educational session. If pretraining competence is tested at 80% to 85% proficiency, posttraining competence might be set at 90% to 95% proficiency. Or, in the patient suicide example described on page 50, measures might include the percentage of accurately and appropriately completed suicide risk assessments as determined through peer review and the percentage of rooms with breakaway shower fixtures.

At times, it may be difficult to establish quantitative measures—the improvement simply seems to lend itself more to qualitative measures. Quantification of improvement is critical, however, and even when solutions can only be measured in terms of risk reduction potential, it is important to try to quantify such potential as much as possible through concrete measures.

Use Worksheet 6-4, page 137, to articulate responses to questions concerning expectations, the sequence of activities, measures, and resources required.

Issue Three: When

Next, the team must define *when* the organization must meet its improvement goals. What time frame will be established for implementing the improvement action? What timeline will be established for each activity comprising the steps along the way? What are the major milestones and their respective dates? A Gantt chart of one organization's improvement plan appears as Figure 6-2, pages 120-121. Use Worksheet 6-5, page 138, to articulate responses to questions concerning time frames and milestones.

 Tool: *Gantt chart*

Issue Four: Who

Who is closest to this process and therefore should "own" the improvement activity? Who should be accountable at various stages? To a great extent, the success of an improvement effort hinges on involving the right people from all disciplines, services, and offices involved in the process being addressed. The process for taking action consists of several stages, each of which may have different players.

The group that creates the process should include the people responsible for the process, the people who carry out the process, and the people affected by the process. As appropriate, the group members could include staff from different units, branch offices or teams, services, disciplines, and job categories. When the group needs a perspective not offered by its representatives, it should conduct interviews or surveys outside the group or invite new members into the group. It is important to consider customers and suppliers such as purchasers, payers, physicians, referral sources, accreditors, regulators, and the community as a whole. *See* Worksheet 6-6, pages 139-140, for more information on key players at each stage.

Leaders and managers must take an active role in overseeing and setting priorities for design and redesign. Generally, managers are responsible for processes within their areas; design or redesign of processes with a wider scope may be overseen by upper management or by a team of managers. Leaders must ensure that the people involved have the necessary resources and expertise. Furthermore, their authority to make changes should be commensurate with their responsibility for process improvements. While regular feedback and contact with management are important, rigid control can stifle creativity.

Issue Five: Where

Where will the improvement action be implemented? Will its implementation be organizationwide, in a selected location, with a selected patient population, or with selected staff members? Are the location, target population, and target staff of the improvement action likely to expand with success? Use Worksheet 6-7, page 141, to indicate where the improvement action will be implemented. Worksheet 6-8, page 142, can be used to provide a summary look at the what, how, when, who, and where involved in implementing proposed improvement actions.

Considering the Impact of Change

When designing improvements, the team should also consider the impact of change on the organization.

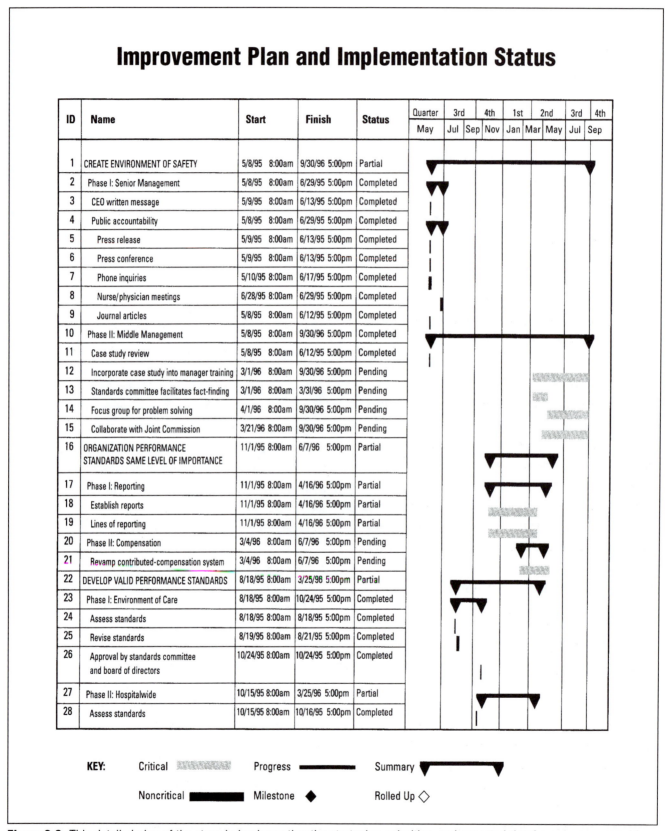

Figure 6-2. This detailed plan of the steps in implementing the strategies, priorities, and expected timeframes was created by an organization following a sentinel event involving a mechanical failure. The status of each phase in the plan is recorded so everyone involved has a clear idea of the progress being made.
Used with permission.

Improvement Plan and Implementation Status, *continued*

ID	Name	Start	Finish	Status	Quarter 3rd — May Jul Sep	4th Nov	1st Jan Mar	2nd May	3rd Jul	4th Sep
29	Revise standards	11/16/95 8:00am	11/24/95 5:00pm	Completed		■				
30	Approval by quality committee and board of directors	2/13/96 8:00am	3/25/96 5:00pm	Partial			▬			
31	HOLD MANAGEMENT ACCOUNTABLE	8/21/95 8:00am	9/27/96 5:00pm	Partial	▼━━━━━━━━━━━━━━━━━━━━━━━▼					
32	Phase I: Flatten the Organization	8/21/95 8:00am	1/19/96 5:00pm	Completed	▬▬▬▬▬					
33	Hunter group assessment	8/21/95 8:00am	11/3/95 5:00pm	Completed	▬▬					
34	Internal assessment	10/2/95 8:00am	12/22/95 5:00pm	Completed	▬▬					
35	Reorganize	1/15/96 8:00am	1/19/96 5:00pm	Completed			▮			
36	Phase II: Revise Management Evaluation	3/4/96 8:00am	9/27/96 5:00pm	Pending			▼━━━━━━━━━━━▼			
37	Criteria: competence, qualifications, performance	3/4/96 8:00am	6/7/96 5:00pm	Pending			▬▬			
38	Assess management competencies	3/4/96 8:00am	9/27/96 5:00pm	Pending			▬▬▬▬▬			
39	System: reward, remedy, termination	3/4/96 8:00am	9/27/96 5:00pm	Pending			▬▬▬▬▬			
40	ENSURE UTILITY SYSTEMS PLANNING	5/8/95 8:00am	9/23/96 5:00pm	Partial	▼━━━━━━━━━━━━━━━━━━━━━━━━━━━━━▼					
41	Phase I: Refine Approach	5/8/95 8:00am	11/1/95 5:00pm	Completed	▬▬▬▬▬					
42	Assess weaknesses	8/1/95 8:00am	8/30/95 5:00pm	Completed	▬					
43	Revise policies	9/1/95 8:00am	10/5/95 5:00pm	Completed	▬					
44	Include participation internal/external	5/8/95 8:00am	11/1/95 5:00pm	Completed	▬▬▬▬▬					
45	Develop prioritization method	8/14/95 8:00am	9/8/95 5:00pm	Completed	▬					
46	Phase II: Evaluate Planning	9/21/96 8:00am	9/23/96 5:00pm	Pending						▮
47	ENSURE ADEQUATE TRAINING	8/14/95 8:00am	3/22/96 5:00pm	Partial	▼━━━━━━━━▼					
48	Phase I: Orientation	8/14/95 8:00am	9/1/95 5:00pm	Completed	▼▼					
49	Review programs	8/14/95 8:00am	8/14/95 5:00pm	Completed	▮					
50	Revise	8/21/95 8:00am	8/21/95 5:00pm	Completed	▮					
51	Deploy	9/1/95 8:00am	9/1/95 5:00pm	Completed	▮					
52	Phase II: Competency Assessment	9/1/95 8:00am	3/15/96 5:00pm	Partial	▼━━━━━━━▼					
53	Implement competency assessment	9/1/95 8:00am	9/1/95 5:00pm	Completed	▮					
54	Evaluate checklist	3/4/96 8:00am	3/8/96 5:00pm	Pending			▮			
55	Refine assessment mechanism	3/11/96 8:00am	3/15/96 5:00pm	Pending			▮			
56	Phase III: Retraining	3/11/96 8:00am	3/22/96 5:00pm	Pending			▼▼			
57	Establish criteria requirements	3/11/96 8:00am	3/15/96 5:00pm	Pending			▮			
58	Establish retraining program	3/18/96 8:00am	3/22/96 5:00pm	Pending			▮			

No matter how minor, improvements require change, and it is normal for individuals and organizations to resist change. Resistance to change can come from inertia, the challenge of managing the change process, the challenge of obtaining necessary knowledge to ensure that the change can be implemented effectively, and resource limitations. The team can identify areas where resistance to change might arise and plan countermeasures using Worksheet 6-9, page 143.

16 Step Sixteen: Ensure Acceptability of the Action Plan

The team has defined the what, how, when, who, and where in an improvement action plan. How does the team know whether it is acceptable to the Joint Commission as part of a root cause analysis in response to a sentinel event?

As mentioned in Chapter 1, an action plan is considered acceptable by the Joint Commission if it does the following:
- Identifies changes that can be implemented to reduce risk, or formulates a rationale for not undertaking such changes
- Where improvement actions are planned, identifies who is responsible for implementation, when the action will be implemented (including any pilot testing), and how the effectiveness of the actions will be evaluated

Checklist 6-2, right, lists the criteria for an acceptable action plan.

17 Step Seventeen: Implement the Improvement Plan

When the goals for improvement have been established, the organization can begin planning and carrying out the improvements. A pilot test implementing improvement on a small scale, monitoring its results, and refining the improvement actions is highly recommended. This enables the team to ensure that the improvement is successful before committing significant organization resources. Pilot testing also aids in building support for the improvement plan, thereby facilitating buy-in by opinion leaders. To pilot test an improvement, the team should follow a systematic method that includes performing Steps 18 through 21 on a limited scale.

A systematic method for design or improvement of processes can help organizations pursue identified opportunities. A standard, yet flexible, process for carrying out these changes should help leaders and others ensure that actions address root causes, involve appropriate people, and result in desired and sustained changes. Depending on an organization's mission and improvement goals, any of the methods described here may be used to implement a process improvement. Three improvement methods are described:
- The scientific method
- The PDSA (plan-do-study-act) cycle
- Critical paths

The Scientific Method

The fundamental components of any improvement process are the following:
- Planning the change
- Testing the change

Checklist 6-2. Criteria for an Acceptable Action Plan

Check to ensure that the action plan has the following attributes:
- ☐ Identifies changes to reduce risk or provides rationale for not undertaking changes
- ☐ Identifies who is responsible for implementation
- ☐ Identifies when action(s) will be implemented
- ☐ Identifies how the effectiveness of action(s) will be evaluated

- Studying its effects
- Implementing changes determined to be worthwhile

Many readers will readily associate the activities listed—plan, test, study, implement—with the scientific method. Indeed, the scientific method is a fundamental, inclusive paradigm for change and includes these steps:
- Determine what is known now (about a process, problem, topic of interest).
- Decide what needs to be learned, changed, or improved.
- Develop a hypothesis about how the change can be accomplished.
- Test the hypothesis.
- Assess the effect of the test. (Compare results of before versus after or traditional versus innovative.)
- Implement successful improvements, or rehypothesize and conduct another experiment.

This orderly, logical, inclusive process for improvement serves organizations well as they attempt to assess and improve performance.

The Plan-Do-Study-Act (PDSA) Cycle

A well-established process for improvement that is based on the scientific method is the PDSA cycle. (This method is also called the PDCA cycle, with the word *check* replacing the word *study*.) This process is attributed to Walter Shewhart, a quality improvement pioneer with Bell Laboratories in the 1920s and 1930s, and is also widely associated with W. Edwards Deming, a student and later a colleague of Shewhart. Deming made the PDCA cycle central to his influential teachings about quality. The cycle is compelling in its logic and simplicity. A brief explanation of this process should help readers not already familiar with the cycle to understand it and its use (*see* Figure 6-3, page 124).

During the *planning* step, an operational plan for testing the chosen improvement action is created. Small-scale testing can help to determine whether the improvement actions are viable, whether they will have the desired result, and whether any refinements are necessary before putting them into full operation. The list of proposed improvement actions should be narrowed to a number that can be reasonably tested—perhaps between two and four, but not often more.

During the planning stage, several issues should be resolved:
- Who will be involved in the test?
- What must they know to participate in the test?
- What are the testing timetables?
- How will the test be implemented?
- Why is the idea being tested?
- What are the success factors?
- How will the process and outcomes of the test be measured and assessed?

The *do* step involves implementing the pilot test and collecting actual performance data.

During the *study* (or *check*) step, data collected during the pilot test are analyzed to determine whether the improvement action was successful in achieving the desired outcomes. To determine the degree of success, actual test performance is compared to desired performance targets and baseline results achieved using the established process.

The next step is the *act* step—to take action. If the pilot test is not successful, the cycle repeats. When actions have been shown to be successful, they are made part of standard operating procedure. The process does not stop here. The effectiveness of the action should continue to be measured and assessed to ensure that improvement is maintained.

The components of the four-step PDSA cycle as they relate to designing and improving processes appear as Checklist 6-3, page 125. A single initiative can involve a number of different testing phases or different change strategies and can therefore require the use of consecutive PDSA cycles.

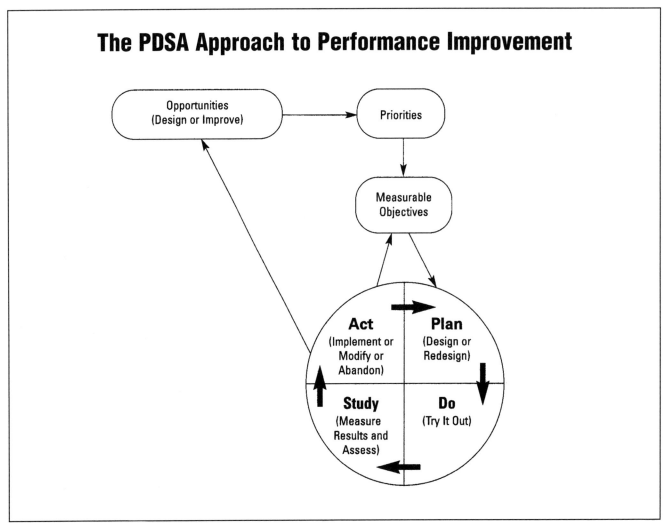

Figure 6-3. The PDSA approach to performance improvement includes identifying design or redesign opportunities, setting priorities for improvement, and implementing the improvement project.

To help teams and individuals involved in design or improvement initiatives apply the method effectively, the organization, depending on the nature of the improvement project, may want to consider the questions outlined in Sidebar 6-3, page 126, at each step of the method.

Critical Paths

One type of process design or redesign that can be used in health care, particularly in response to a sentinel event in a hospital setting, is the development of a critical path (also referred to as a clinical path and clinical or critical pathway). The primary objective of critical pathways is to reduce common-cause variation, thereby reducing the risk of special-cause variation (sentinel events) in dependent processes. Critical paths offer a systematic, flexible guide for standardization of patient care that can start, for example, before admission and follow the patient across all care settings. They are designed by those involved in the process—clients, clinicians, nurses, pharmacists, and others—who come together to offer their unique perspectives and expertise.

A critical path is an excellent way to redesign an existing clinical process that needs change. One advantage of a critical path is the opportunity to start fresh, cast aside traditional but not particularly

> ### Checklist 6-3. Components of the PDSA Cycle
>
> **Plan**
> - ☐ Develop or design a new process, or redesign or improve an existing process.
> - ☐ Determine how to test the new or redesigned process.
> - ☐ Identify measures that can be used to assess the success of the strategy and whether the objective was reached.
> - ☐ Determine how to collect measures of success (MOS).
> - ☐ Involve the right people in development and testing.
>
> **Do**
> - ☐ Run the test of the new or redesigned process, preferably on a small scale.
> - ☐ Collect data on the MOS.
>
> **Study**
> - ☐ Assess the results of the test.
> - ☐ Determine whether the change was successful.
> - ☐ Identify any lessons learned.
>
> **Act**
> - ☐ Implement the change permanently;
> - ☐ Modify it and run it through another testing cycle; or
> - ☐ Abandon it and develop a new approach to test.

effective procedures, and research and implement the best practices. Many critical paths have been developed to date by numerous organizations, including professional societies, government agencies, and health care organizations. These may provide guidance.

A summary of the steps involved in critical path development and implementation appears as Sidebar 6-4, page 127.

Additional Improvement Tools

The following tools are useful for taking action to improve processes:

- *Brainstorming* can be used to create ideas for improvement actions.
- *Multivoting* and *selection grids* can help a team decide between possible improvement actions.
- *Flowcharts* can help a team understand the current process and how the new or redesigned process should work.
- *Cause-and-effect diagrams* can indicate which changes might cause the desired result or goal.
- *Pareto charts* can help determine which changes are likely to have the greatest effect in reaching the goal.
- *Run charts, control charts, line graphs, pie graphs,* and *scatter diagrams* can measure the effect of a process change or variation in processes and outcomes.
- *Histograms* and *data tables* can show how much effect each change has had.

Tools: *Brainstorming, multivoting, selection grid, flowchart, cause-and-effect diagram, Pareto chart, run chart, control chart, histogram, line graph, pie graph, scatter diagram, data table*

Creating and Managing the Change

Some suggested actions the team might take to help manage and lead the change or improvement process follow.[9] These are based on eight sequential stages in the process of leading change in organizations.[10] The steps in creating and managing the change process are as follows:

1. Establish a sense of urgency by doing the following:
   - Identifying the best anywhere and the gap between one process and another

Sidebar 6-3. Key Questions to Consider During the PDSA Cycle

Plan:
- How was a design or improvement strategy selected for testing?
- Is there knowledge-based information (for example, from the literature, other organizations, or other external sources) supporting the new or improved process?
- What issues in the external environment (such as economy, politics, customer needs, competitors, regulations) will affect the performance of the new or improved process?
- What issues in the internal environment will affect the performance of the new or improved process?
- Who is (are) the customer(s) of the process?
- What is the current process?
- What is the desired process?
- Who are the suppliers of the process?
- What changes will have the most impact?
- Is there a plan for testing the design or improvement?
- Is there a timeline for testing?
- What data will be collected to determine whether the test was successful (that is, whether the objective was met)?
- How is it determined that the measures actually address the desired issue?
- Can the measures used actually track performance?
- How will data be collected?
- Who will collect data?
- Are systems in place to support planned measurement?
- Is benchmarking feasible for this initiative?
- Are the right people involved?
- What resources are needed to design or redesign the process? What resources are available?

Do:
- Was the testing plan followed?
- Were needed modifications discussed with the appropriate people?
- Was data collection timely?
- Was data collection reliable?

Study:
- How will the test data be assessed?
- What process should be used?
- Who should be involved in data analysis?
- What methods or tools should we use to analyze data?
- Is training needed on data analysis methods and tools?
- Is comparative data (internal or external) available?
- Does data analysis lead to an understanding of problem areas?
- Are data analyses timely? Are the results available soon enough to take needed actions?
- Did the test data indicate that the design or improvement was successful?
- What lessons were learned from the test?
- What measures will determine whether to implement the tested design or improvement on a permanent basis?
- How and to whom will the results of assessment activities be communicated?

Act:
- Should changes be recommended to others (for example, for purchasing equipment or implementing specific processes)?
- How will these changes be communicated to the appropriate people?
- Is any education or training needed?
- How will gain be maintained and backsliding be prevented?
- What measures should be used to assess the performance of the new or improved product or process?
- Should any of the measures identified previously be included in ongoing measurement activities?

Sidebar 6-4. Developing and Implementing a Critical Path

Selecting the Process
The initial step in creating a critical path is choosing a process to standardize. The first part of the root cause analysis identifies the relevant process(es) that requires redesign. The time needed to develop a critical path may vary from two hours to four months.[1] Organizations should be prepared for a significant commitment of time.

Defining the Diagnosis, Condition, or Procedure
An appropriately defined process and patient population simplifies critical path development. A process that is too broadly defined results in a path that is either too complex or too vague; conversely, a process that is too narrowly defined can result in a path that applies in only a limited number of cases.[2,3]

Forming a Team
The group that creates the critical path must represent all disciplines involved in the process. The scope of the process helps determine team members. Another valuable perspective comes from patients and their families or caregivers, customers, and others. The team should elicit information from the people the process is designed to benefit. Similarly, if other parties are involved but are not team members, their input must also be elicited.

Identifying or Creating the Critical Path
Team members must reach consensus on the key activities involved in each stage of the care process. Members can draw on personal experience and knowledge, existing clinical literature and practice guidelines, and patient perspectives. When varying styles or methods of care arise—as they inevitably will—the team should not panic. The resulting discussion can yield important knowledge about patient care. If varied practice patterns are such that the group cannot reach consensus, the path should not dictate one approach over another; separate paths can be developed when necessary.[3] Subsequent outcome measurement may demonstrate an advantage of one path over another. The path need not be limited to clinical activities; it can also include activities that surround the clinical process, such as transportation to the radiology department. Critical paths should also include descriptions of expected outcomes. Despite the complexity of the processes involved, teams should attempt to make their paths as concise as possible—one page is ideal—so they can be used as practical tools in daily practice.

Results
At all stages of the care process, organization staff can refer to critical paths. They should be available to all involved personnel in all relevant work areas and office locations. Critical paths are also valuable for patients; they can increase patients' knowledge and sense of partnership with providers.[1-3]

References
1. Weber D.O.: Clinical pathways stretch patient care but shrink costly lengths of stay at Anne Arundel Medical Center in Annapolis, Maryland. *Strategic Health Excell* 5(5):1–9, 1992.
2. Bower K.A.: Developing and using critical paths. Lord J.T. (ed.): *The Physician Leader's Guide*. Rockville, MD: Bader & Associates, Inc., 1992, pp. 61–66.
3. Zander K.: Critical pathways. Melum M.M., Sinioris M.K. (eds.): *Total Quality Management*: The Health Care Pioneers. Chicago: American Hospital Publishing, Inc., 1992, pp. 305–314.

- Identifying the consequence of being less than the best
- Exploring sources of complacency

2. Create a guiding coalition to do the following:
   - Find the right people
   - Create trust
   - Share a common goal

3. Develop a vision and strategy that is the following:
   - Easily pictured
   - Attractive
   - Feasible and clear
   - Flexible
   - Communicable

4. Communicate the changed vision in a way that does the following:
   - Is simple
   - Uses metaphor
   - Works in multiple forms
   - Involves doing instead of telling
   - Explains inconsistencies
   - Involves give and take

5. Empower broad-based action by doing the following:
   - Communicating sensible vision to employees
   - Making organization structures compatible with action
   - Providing needed training
   - Aligning information and human resource systems
   - Confronting supervisors who undercut change

6. Generate short-term wins by the following:
   - Fixing the date of certain change
   - Doing the easy stuff first
   - Using measurement to confirm change

7. Consolidate gains and produce more change by doing the following:
   - Identifying true interdependencies and smooth interconnections
   - Eliminating unnecessary dependencies
   - Identifying linked subsequent cycles of change

8. Anchor new approaches in the culture with the following:
   - Results
   - Conversation
   - Turnover
   - Succession

18 Step Eighteen: Develop Measures of Effectiveness and Ensure Their Success

Previous pages described how to design or redesign a function or process where the improvement cycle often begins. When a function or process is underway, the team should collect data about its performance. As described in Chapter 4, measurement is the process of collecting and aggregating these data, a process that helps assess the level of performance and determine whether further improvement actions are necessary. Specifically, measurement can be used as an integral technique throughout the PDSA cycle to do the following:

- Assist in process design or redesign (the plan step)
- Test whether process design or redesign is implemented properly (the do step)
- Assess the results of the test (the study step)
- Provide assistance in implementing the improvement (the act step)
- Maintain the improvement and determine whether the improvement should be part of the organization's ongoing monitoring process (repeat of the PDSA cycle)

A description of each use appears in Chapter 4, pages 82-85. This discussion focuses on measurement's use to determine whether improvement has occurred and is sustained.

The first step in measuring the success of improvement efforts is to develop high-quality measures of effectiveness. The choice of what to measure is critical. Measurement must relate to the improvement and validate the accomplishment of the goal (or failure to reach the goal). See Checklist 4-1, page 85, for a list of key criteria for measures, and Sidebar 4-3, page 85, for key questions the team should ask concerning what to measure. Answer the questions in Worksheet 6-10, pages 144-145, as the team identifies, measures, and designs the measurement plan.

Some measures or performance indicators may require specific targets, and these should be set by the team prior to data collection. For example, in the patient suicide case described on page 50, the team should set 100% as the target for bringing rooms in the behavioral health unit into compliance with breakaway shower fixtures. For the treatment delay example, the team should set a score of 95% as the target for all post-training test scores. Data collection efforts should be planned and coordinated. Use a separate worksheet to plan and monitor the indicators selected to measure each improvement goal (*see* Worksheet 6-11, page 146). Use Checklist 6-4, right, to help ensure that the team has considered important attributes of measurement success.

Who should be responsible for measurement? The team, empowered to study the process and recommend changes, is usually responsible for designing and carrying out the measurement activities necessary to determine how the process performs. After making changes to improve the process, the team should continue to apply some or all its measures to determine whether the change has had the desired effect. Organizations may have various experts who can help design measurement activities, including experts in information management, quality improvement, and the function to be measured. The team can request such contribution on an ad hoc basis. For example, if the team is investigating a medication error and has a large amount of data to codify and process regarding the administration of a frequently ordered drug, the team may want to seek the help of information management staff with access to statistical software capable of analyzing a large volume of data.

Checklist 6-4. Assuring the Success of Measurement

An affirmative answer to the following questions gives the team a good indication that it is on the right track with its efforts to measure the effectiveness of improvement initiatives.

Yes   No
☐   ☐   Is there a plan for use of the data?
☐   ☐   Are the data collected reliable and valid?
☐   ☐   Has ease of data collection been assured?
☐   ☐   Have key elements required for improvement been defined?
☐   ☐   Has a data rich–information poor syndrome been avoided?
☐   ☐   Has a key point for information dissemination been designated?

Tip: Avoid Data Collection Redundancy
Make every effort to coordinate any ongoing measurement with data collection already taking place as part of the organization's everyday activities.

Information management professionals and those responsible for carrying out the process being measured are key players in data collection and analysis. The people involved vary widely depending on the specific organization, the function being measured, and the measurement process.

Step Nineteen: Evaluate Implementation of Improvement Efforts

After data are collected as part of measurement, they must be translated into information that the team can use to make judgments and draw conclusions about the performance of improvement efforts. This assessment forms the basis for further actions taken with improvement initiatives.

Numerous techniques can be used to assess the data collected. Most types of assessment require comparing data to a point of reference. These reference points may include the following:
- Internal comparisons
- Aggregate external reference databases
- Practice guidelines/parameters
- Desired performance targets, specifications, or thresholds

Internal Comparisons
The team can compare its current performance with its past performance using statistical quality control tools. Three such tools are especially helpful in comparing performance with historical patterns and assessing variation and stability: run charts, control charts, and histograms. These show changes over time, variation in performance, and the stability of performance.

Tools: Run chart, control chart, histogram

Aggregate External Reference Databases
In addition to assessing the organization's own historical patterns of performance, the team can compare the organization's performance with that of other organizations. Expanding the scope of comparison helps an organization draw conclusions about its own performance and learn about different methods to design and carry out processes. Aggregate external databases take various forms. Aggregate, risk-adjusted data about specific indicators help each organization set priorities for improvement by showing whether its current performance falls within the expected range.

One method of comparing performance is *benchmarking*. Although a benchmark can be any point of comparison, most often it is a standard of excellence. Benchmarking is the process by which one organization studies the exemplary performance of a similar process in another organization and, to the greatest extent possible, adapts that information for its own use. Or the team may wish to simply compare its results with those of other organizations or with current research or literature.

Assessment is not confined to information gathered within the walls of a single organization. To better understand its level of performance, an organization should compare its performance against reference databases, professional standards, trade association guidelines, and other sources.

Practice Guidelines or Parameters
Practice guidelines or parameters, critical paths, and other standardized patient care procedures are very useful reference points for comparison. Whether developed by professional societies or in-house practitioners, these procedures represent an expert consensus about the expected practices for a given diagnosis or treatment. Assessing variation from such established procedures can help the team identify how to improve a process.

Desired Performance Targets
The team may also establish targets, specifications, or thresholds for evaluation against which to compare current performance. Such levels can be derived from professional literature or expert opinion within the organization.

Step Twenty: Take Additional Action

The team's assessment of the data collected indicates whether established targets or goals are being achieved. If the goals are being

achieved, the team's efforts now should focus on communicating, standardizing, and rolling out the successful improvement initiatives. The team can do the following:
- Communicate the results, as described in Step 21, below.
- Revise processes and procedures so that the improvement is realized in everyday work.
- Complete necessary training so that all staff are up to speed on the new process or procedure.
- Establish a plan to monitor the improvement's ongoing effectiveness.
- Identify other areas where the improvement could be rolled out.

Organizations frequently falter when continued measurement indicates that improvement goals are not being sustained. Efforts tend, more often than not, to provide short-term rather than long-term improvement. If the team is not achieving the improvement goals, it needs to revisit the improvement actions by circling back to confirm root causes, identify a risk reduction strategy, design an improvement, implement an action plan, and measure the effectiveness of that plan over time.

There are a number of reasons a team's improvements may falter and fail.[11] If the team is having trouble effecting improvement, consider the reasons and remedies shown in Sidebar 6-5, page 132.

Step Twenty-One: Communicate the Results

21

Throughout the root cause analysis process, the team should be communicating team conclusions and recommendations as outlined by the team early in the process (*see* Chapter 3, pages 59 and 61). Hence, the communication process occurs throughout the team's effort and is critical to the success of improvement initiatives.

After determining what happened or could have happened and identifying root causes of the event or possible event, the team should provide leadership with the recommendations for improvement actions to prevent a recurrence of the event. Generally, a short written report provides leaders with the summary they need. An outline of the contents of such a report appears as Sidebar 6-6, page 133. The team should consider with care how and to whom the report is to be presented. Participants during a formal oral presentation should include those whose approval and help is needed, as well as those who could gain from the team's recommendations. Consider the following questions in communicating an improvement initiative:

- How will implementation of this initiative be communicated throughout the organization? Who needs to know?
- What communication vehicles will the team use for various audiences (individuals both directly and indirectly affected by the improvement)?

Following implementation of such actions and measuring and assuring their success, the team should report to leadership on the results of the improvement actions. The report should include information regarding applicability to other processes, areas, and locations and the lessons learned.

References

1. Leape L.L.: Error in medicine. *JAMA* 272(23):1855, 1994.
2. Moray N.: Error reduction as a systems problem. In Bogner M.S. (ed.): *Human Error in Medicine.* Hillsdale, NJ: Lawrence Erlbaum Associates, 1994, pp. 70–71.
3. Leape, p. 1854.
4. Joint Commission: *Failure Mode and Effects Analysis (FMEA): Proactive Risk Reduction, Second Edition.* Oakbrook Terrace, IL: Joint Commission on Accreditation of Healthcare Organizations, 2005.
5. Fletcher C.E.: Failure mode and effects analysis: An interdisciplinary way to analyze and reduce medication errors. *J Nurs Adm* 27(12):19–26, 1997.
6. Wilson P.F., Dell L.D., Anderson G.F.: *Root Cause Analysis: A Tool for Total Quality Management.* Milwaukee: ASQC Quality Press, 1993, p. 75.
7. Spath P.L.: *Investigating Sentinel Events: How to Find and Resolve Root Causes.* Forest Grove, OR: Brown-Spath & Associates, 1997, pp. 107–108.

> **Sidebar 6-5. When Improvements Falter: Reasons and Remedies**
>
> **Problem**
> - Failure to hold the gains because the improvement required major changes
> - Failure to hold the gains because the improvement created extra work or hassle
> - Failure to hold the gains because new staff or leadership were not trained in the improved process
> - Inability to replicate in other settings
> - Not enough public or personal attention to improvement success
> - Inadequate institutional and administrative support
> - Hidden barriers to needed changes
> - A cookie-cutter approach to replicating improvement
>
> **Remedy**
> - Big changes are best arrived at one step at a time.
> - Design improvements so the desired task is the easiest thing do. Design a robust process that makes it easy to do things right and difficult to do things incorrectly.
> - Ensure continued training of all appropriate staff.
> - Build a lasting improvement by recognizing that individuals adopt innovations after passing through a series of stages, including knowledge (becoming aware that a new idea exists), persuasion (forming a favorable attitude toward the new idea), decision (choosing to adopt the innovation), implementation (putting the idea into use), and confirmation (seeking further confirmation about the innovation leading to either continued adoption or discontinuance). Consider and plan for this process when bringing an improvement to each and every setting.
> - Leaders must ensure that improvement successes are recognized and celebrated.
> - Leaders must provide time and talent.
> - Leaders must empower improvement teams to identify where changes are needed and help them make the changes happen.
> - Process improvements must be reinvented at each new site, adapted to meet local circumstances, and fingerprinted by the local owners of the newly improved press.

Source: James B.C., Ryer J.: Holding the gains. Nelson E.C., Batalden P.B., Ryer J. (eds.): *Clinical Improvement Action Guide*. Oakbrook Terrace, IL: Joint Commission on Accreditation of Healthcare Organizations, 1998, pp. 121–124.

8. Ammerman M.: *The Root Cause Analysis Handbook: A Simplified Approach to Identifying, Correcting, and Reporting Workplace Errors.* New York: Quality Resources, 1998, p. 73.
9. Nelson E.C., Batalden P.B., Ryer J. (eds.): *Clinical Improvement Action Guide.* Oakbrook Terrace, IL: Joint Commission, 1998, pp. 116–117.
10. Kotter J.P.: *Leading Change.* Boston: Harvard Business School Press, 1996.
11. James B.C., Ryer J.: Holding the gains. Nelson E.C., Batalden P.B., Ryer J. (eds.): *Clinical Improvement Action Guide.* Oakbrook Terrace, IL: Joint Commission on Accreditation of Healthcare Organizations, 1998, pp. 121–124.

Sidebar 6-6. Possible Content of Report to Leaders

Event Description
This section includes a brief description of the sentinel event or possible event. It includes what, when, where, who, and how information as articulated in the problem definition (*see* Chapter 3, pages 55-57). The emphasis is on facts related to the event and the areas involved.

Scope of Analysis
This section describes the team's membership and purpose, and the analytical methods used to investigate the event or possible event.

Proximate Causes and Immediate Responses
This section describes the circumstances leading to the event, proximate causes identified by the team, and any response strategies and corrective actions implemented by individuals immediately following the event.

Root Causes
This section describes the analyses conducted to determine root causes and lists the root causes identified by the team.

Improvement Actions and Follow-Up Plan
This section describes the improvement actions recommended by the team for each root cause. It also describes the measures and time frame recommended to evaluate the effectiveness of improvement actions.

Worksheet 6-1. Prioritizing Improvement Actions

Use the following worksheet to catalog improvement actions suggested by the team. Separate sheets for each root cause and its suggested improvement actions may be used. The team should also rate or rank improvement actions based on agreed-upon criteria. Use this worksheet to record the rankings of individual team members and the team as a whole.

Root Causes	Suggested Improvement Actions	Ranking
Root Cause 1: _____	_____	_____
_____	_____	_____
_____	_____	_____
_____	_____	_____
_____	_____	_____
Root Cause 2: _____	_____	_____
_____	_____	_____
_____	_____	_____
_____	_____	_____
_____	_____	_____
Root Cause 3: _____	_____	_____
_____	_____	_____
_____	_____	_____
_____	_____	_____
_____	_____	_____

Worksheet 6-2. Summarizing the Potential of Improvement Actions

Two questions help the team summarize the potential of each proposed improvement action. Use the space following each question to provide a concise answer.

What will result from implementing this action?

_____
_____
_____
_____
_____
_____
_____
_____

What would result from not implementing this action?

_____
_____
_____
_____
_____
_____
_____
_____

Worksheet 6-3. Defining Improvement Goals, Scope, and Activities

This worksheet helps the team define what it is trying to improve. Use the space following each question to provide as concise an answer as possible.

What goals does the organization have in implementing necessary improvements related to a sentinel event or possible event?

_____
_____
_____
_____

What dimensions of performance will be most affected by the change?

_____
_____
_____
_____

What specific activities must be carried out to reach the goals and affect the dimensions of performance? (Provide a clear statement of the essential features of each proposed solution.) What are the sequential steps necessary to accomplish the proposed improvement?

1. _____
2. _____
3. _____
4. _____
5. _____
6. _____

Worksheet 6-4. Defining Improvement Expectations, Sequence, Resources, and Measures

This worksheet helps the team define how the organization will meet its improvement goals. Use the space following each question to provide as concise an answer as possible.

How must the improved process perform?

_____
_____
_____

What sequence of activities will be required to meet these expectations?

_____
_____
_____

What resources will be required to meet these expectations?

_____
_____
_____

How and what will be measured to determine whether the process is actually performing at the level expected?

Improvement Action	Quantitative Measure

Worksheet 6-5. Defining Time Frames and Milestones

This worksheet helps the team define when the organization will meet its improvement goals. Use the space following each question to provide as concise an answer as possible.

What time frame will be established for implementing the overall improvement action?

_____
_____
_____
_____
_____

What timeline will be established for each activity comprising the steps along the way?

Activity   **Time frame**

_____
_____
_____
_____
_____

What are the major milestones and their respective completion dates?

Milestone   **Completion date**

_____
_____
_____
_____
_____

Worksheet 6-6. Involving the Right People

Involving the right people at each stage of the improvement process is critical to the success of the improvement initiative. Consider which individuals should be involved at each stage, and write their names in the appropriate spaces.

Designing the action. In general, the group that participated in the root cause analysis should have the necessary expertise to recommend improvements and may be in the best position to design or redesign the improvements. This group should include those who carry out or are affected by the process. They are

_____

_____

_____

_____

_____

_____

Approving recommended actions. When substantial resources are involved and the potential effects are significant, the organization's leaders usually have to approve the action. This is most certainly the case with improvements recommended following a sentinel event. If a group has obtained the necessary input and buy-in while devising an improvement, the approval should come readily. The appropriate leaders are

_____

_____

_____

_____

_____

_____

Worksheet 6-6. Involving the Right People, *continued*

Testing the action. Testing should occur under real world conditions, involving staff who will actually be carrying out the process. Effects can be measured with the same methods used to establish a performance baseline. Appropriate staff members include

___

___

___

___

___

___

___

Implementing the action. Although full-scale implementation of a process change should have positive results, any change can create anxiety. Therefore, care should be taken to prepare people for change and to explain the reason for the change in an educational, nonthreatening way. Cooperation is essential for changes to succeed, but cannot exist if people believe a change is being forced on them without good reason. An effective team should have already acquired much of the necessary buy-in during earlier phases of the improvement process or during the early stages in the root cause analysis. Appropriate staff members include

___

___

___

___

___

___

___

Worksheet 6-7. Determining Location of Improvement Actions

This worksheet helps the team define where the organization will implement improvement goals.

Where will the improvement action be implemented?

_____
_____
_____
_____

Will its implementation be organizationwide or in a selected location with a selected patient population or selected staff members?

_____
_____
_____
_____

Are the location, target population, and target staff of the improvement action likely to expand with success?

☐ No (If no, why not?) ☐ Yes (If yes, how?)

_____
_____
_____
_____

Worksheet 6-8. Integrating the Improvement Plan

Define the timelines and responsibilities associated with each of the project steps using the following table. (Customize column headers as desired.) Questions to consider include the following:
- What are the timelines for each step of the project and for the project as a whole?
- What will be the checkpoints, control points, or milestones for project assessment?
- Who is responsible for each step or milestone?
- Who is responsible for corrective course action?
- What staff members will be involved in the improvement project?
- What will be the nature and extent of their responsibilities?

Steps to Be Taken	Date of Implementation	Areas for Implementation	Individuals Responsible	Other Considerations

Worksheet 6-9. Identifying Change Barriers and Solutions

Use this worksheet to identify possible barriers to change and solutions to overcome such barriers.

Areas where resistance to change might emerge include

_____
_____
_____
_____
_____
_____
_____
_____
_____

Countermeasures to overcome such barriers include

_____
_____
_____
_____
_____
_____
_____
_____
_____
_____

Worksheet 6-10. Designing the Measurement Plan

What is the scope of measurement for the improvement project?
_____
_____

Have any portions of the process under study been measured in the past, or are they currently being measured? If so, are assessments available?
_____
_____

What measurement tools will be used for this initiative?
_____
_____

Will the tools provide reliable data? Have they been tested?
_____
_____

What costs are associated with collecting the necessary data? Do benefits outweigh costs?
_____
_____

Can the data generated by the selected measurement tool be transformed into meaningful and useful information?
_____
_____

How can the team ensure that the data are complete, accurate, and unbiased?
_____
_____

Worksheet 6-10. Designing the Measurement Plan, *continued*

How will the staff collecting data be educated?

_____
_____
_____
_____

What format(s) will be used to report the data?

_____
_____
_____
_____

Where and how will any additional data needed be obtained?

_____
_____
_____
_____

How will the success of the improvement be measured?

_____
_____
_____
_____

Source: Adapted from Hanold L.S., Vinson B.E., Rubino A.: Evaluating and improving the medication use system. Cousins D.D. (ed.): *Medication Use: A Systems Approach to Reducing Errors*. Oakbrook Terrace, IL: Joint Commission on Accreditation of Healthcare Organizations, 1998, pp. 93–96.

Worksheet 6-11. Evaluating Target Goals

Use a worksheet like this one to plan and monitor progress in measuring the effectiveness of each improvement goal.

Goal	Measure	Person Responsible	Review Completed

Chapter 7
Tools and Techniques

This chapter provides information on selected tools and techniques that can be used during root cause analysis. The tools and techniques are presented in a uniform format, or profile, to assist readers with their selection and use. *Profiles* identify the stage of root cause analysis during which the tool or technique may be used, its purpose, simple usage steps, and tips for effective use. An example of the tool or technique follows each profile.

When embarking on a root cause analysis, team members may wish to start by consulting the tool matrix appearing as Figure 7-1, page 148. This matrix lists many of the tools and techniques available during root cause analysis and indicates the stages during which they may be particularly helpful. Not all the tools listed in the matrix are profiled in this chapter. For additional information on specific tools and techniques, readers are advised to consult the Bibliography, which contains references to many excellent monographs and workbooks.

Tool Profile:
Affinity Diagram
(See Figure 7-2, page 149)

Stages to Use: Identifying proximate causes; identifying root causes; identifying improvement opportunities

Purpose: To creatively generate a large volume of ideas or issues and then organize them into meaningful groups.

Simple Steps to Success:
1. Choose a team.
2. Define the issue in the broadest and most neutral manner.
3. Brainstorm the issue and record the ideas.
4. Randomly display cards or notes with the ideas so that everyone can see them.
5. Sort the ideas into groups of related topics.
6. Create header or title cards for each grouping.
7. Draw the diagram, connecting all header cards with their groupings.

Tips for Effective Use
- Keep the team small (four to six people) and ensure varied perspectives.
- Generate as many ideas as possible using brainstorming guidelines.
- Record ideas from brainstorming on index cards or adhesive notes.
- Sort the ideas in silence, being guided in sorting only by gut instinct.
- If an idea keeps getting moved back and forth from one group to another, agree to create a duplicate card or note.
- Reach a consensus on how cards are sorted.
- Allow some ideas to stand alone.
- Make sure that each idea has at least a noun and a verb when appropriate; avoid using single words.
- Break large groupings into subgroups with subtitles, but be careful not to slow progress with too much definition.

Tool Matrix

Tools	Proximate	Root	Identifying Improvements	Implementing and Monitoring Improvements
Affinity diagram	x	x	x	
Barrier analysis	x			x
Box plot		x		
Brainstorming	x		x	
Cause-and-effect diagram	x	x		
Change analysis	x			
Check sheets		x		x
Contingency diagram	x		x	x
Control charts		x	x	x
Cost-of-quality analysis	x			
Critical-to-quality analysis	x			
Decision matrix		x	x	
Deployment flowchart	x		x	x
Effective-achievable matrix		x	x	
Failure mode and effects analysis (FMEA)			x	
Fault tree analysis	x	x	x	
Fishbone diagram	x	x		
Flowchart	x	x	x	x
Force field analysis	x		x	x
Gantt chart	x	x	x	x
Graphs		x		x
Histogram	x	x	x	x
Ishikawa diagram	x	x		
Is–is not matrix		x		
Kolmogorov-Smirnov test		x		x
List reduction		x	x	
Matrix diagram		x	x	x
Multivoting	x	x	x	
Nominal group technique (NGT)	x		x	
Normal probability plot		x		x
Operational definitions		x	x	x
Pareto chart		x	x	
PDSA (plan-do-study-act) cycle				x
PMI (plus, minus, interesting)		x	x	
Relations diagram	x	x	x	
Run chart	x	x		x
Scatter diagram (scattergram)		x		x
Storyboard			x	x
Stratification		x		
Timeline	x	x		
Top-down flowchart	x		x	x
Why-why diagram	x			
Work-flow diagram	x		x	x

Figure 7-1. This matrix lists many of the tools and techniques available during root cause analysis and indicates the stages during which they may be particularly helpful. Not all the tools are profiled in this chapter.

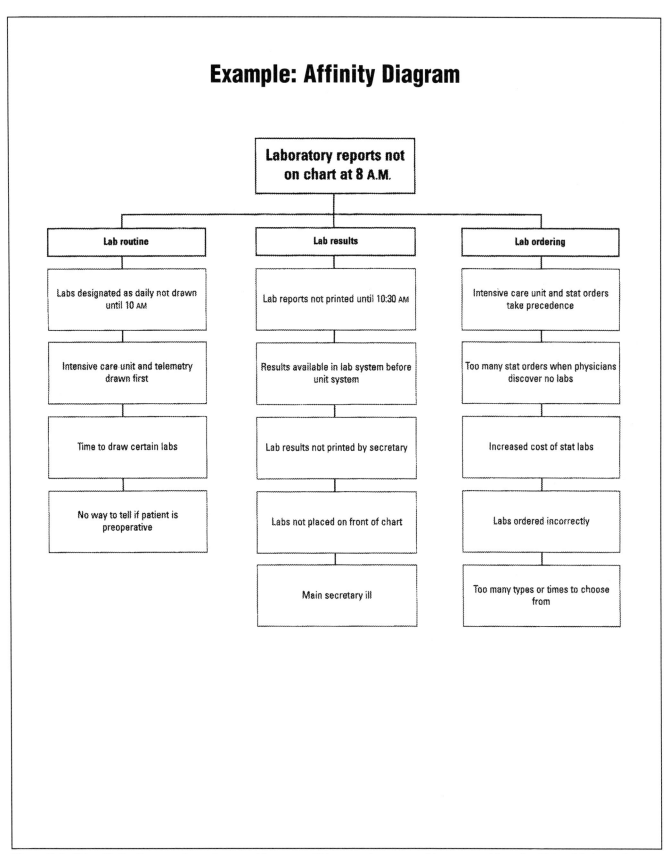

Figure 7-2. This affinity diagram shows how a wide range of ideas can be arranged in manageable order. Using this type of diagram presents ideas on why laboratory results are not available as needed in three categories: routine, results, and ordering.

Tool Profile:
Barrier Analysis
(See Figure 7-3, page 151)

Stages to Use: Identifying proximate causes; implementing and monitoring improvements

Purpose: To offer a structured way of visualizing the events related to system failure or the creation of a problem. It can be used reactively to solve problems, investigate sentinel events, or identify missing safeguards or proactively to evaluate existing barriers or identify additional barriers that should be considered to prevent recurrence of unwanted events.

Simple Steps to Success:
1. Define the targets. *Targets* are those things of value that can be harmed by threats. Identify what has been damaged or could have been damaged by the threat.
2. Identify the threat. *Threats* are those hazards or potential problems that cause harm or an adverse outcome or have the potential to do so.
3. Identify the barriers. *Barriers* are those things that should have prevented or could prevent the undesired event.
4. Analyze the barriers. This involves analyzing the adequacy of the barriers by asking questions about their performance.
5. Identify apparent or proximate causes and the root cause. List all the proximate causes and root cause(s).
6. Devise and recommend corrective or preventive actions.

Tips for Effective Use
- Remember that the list of targets may include multiple items.
- Be aware that with sentinel events occurring in health care facilities, targets are generally the people, either individually or collectively, who can be damaged or harmed by an unwanted incident. However, targets can also be material things such as buildings and equipment; nonmaterial things such as goodwill, friendship, and status; or the environment.
- List all the potential targets initially and let follow-up analysis eliminate those not affected by the event.
- To analyze the barriers, ask the questions, "Were barriers in place to minimize threats to the target? Were such barriers adequate? That is, were they capable of handling the threat? Were there backups for each barrier?"
- Be aware that each less-than-adequate barrier can be attributed to a different proximate cause.
- The root cause can be identified as the cause that appears most often in explaining inadequate barriers or the cause that, if eliminated, would preclude the event from happening.
- Use a simple worksheet to record the barrier analysis.

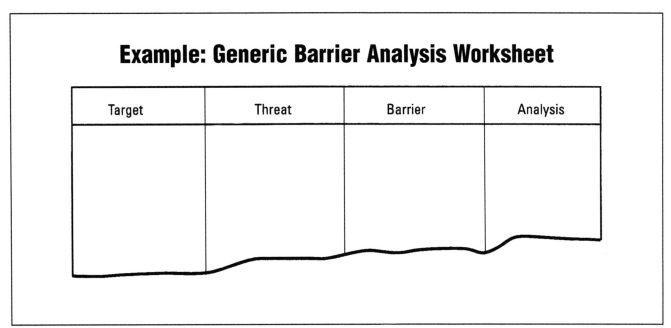

Figure 7-3. This generic worksheet shows a simple way of listing and comparing information for barrier analysis. The worksheet is arranged in columns to lead logically from the target to threat(s), barrier(s), and analysis.
Source: Wilson P.F., Dell L.D., Anderson G.F.: *Root Cause Analysis: A Tool for Total Quality Management*. Milwaukee: ASQC Quality Press, 1993, p. 147. Used with permission.

Tool Profile:
Brainstorming
(See Figure 7-4, page 153)

Stages to Use: Identifying proximate causes; identifying improvement opportunities

Purpose: To generate multiple ideas in a minimum amount of time through a creative group process.

Simple Steps to Success:
1. Define the subject. This ensures that the session has direction.
2. Think briefly about the issue. Allow enough time for team members to gather their thoughts, but not enough time for detailed analysis.
3. Set a time limit. There should be enough time for every member to make a contribution, but keep it short to prevent premature analysis of ideas.
4. Generate ideas. Use a structured format where the group members express ideas by taking turns in a predetermined order and the process continues in rotation until either time runs out or ideas are exhausted, or use an unstructured format where group members voice ideas as they come to mind.
5. Clarify ideas. The goal is to make sure that all ideas are recorded accurately and are understood by the group.

Tips for Effective Use
- Create a nonthreatening, safe environment for expressing ideas.
- Tell the group upfront that any idea is welcome, no matter how narrow or broad in scope, how serious or light in nature. All ideas are valuable, as long as they address the subject at hand.
- Remember that the best ideas are sometimes the most unusual.
- Never criticize ideas. It is crucial that neither the leader nor the other group members comment on any given idea.
- In thinking briefly about the issue (step 2), do not give group members time to second-guess their ideas. Be aware that self-censorship stifles creative thought.
- Write down all ideas on a chalkboard or easel so that the group can view them.
- Keep it short; enforce a time limit of 10 to 20 minutes.
- In organizations where staff may not regularly be in a centralized location, brainstorming can be done by asking staff to submit as many ideas as possible about the topic in writing, by voice mail, or by electronic mail.
- Limit brainstorming to one "level" at a time. For example, when brainstorming possible causes for miscommunication of patient information identified as contributing to the proximate cause of a medication error, teams should hold off on exploring deeper causes such as organization culture and leadership issues.
- Note deeper root causes that emerge during brainstorming in a "parking lot" list for consideration later.

Example: Brainstorming List

Possible causes of a surgical error include the following:
- No timely case review
- No mechanism to ensure patient identity
- Informal case referral process
- Untimely operative dictation
- Inadequate presurgical evaluation
- No review of patient care information prior to surgery
- Inadequate informed consent
- Patient care information unavailable for preoperative review
- Failure to perform surgery in a safe manner
- Laterality not clearly identified
- Delay in reporting of incident
- No multidisciplinary review
- Ignored pathology reports
- History of inadequate documentation in medical record
- Procedures performed without adequate expertise
- Failure to take responsibility for actions and
- No surgical plan/preoperative findings

Figure 7-4. This figure shows an excerpt from a list one organization created using brainstorming to identify possible causes of a surgical error. This list was used to create the cause-and-effect diagram that appears as Figure 7-5, page 155. As the example shows, the ideas are widely varied, and some seem more viable than others. This is intended: brainstorming is for generating ideas, not sorting or judging them.

Root Cause Analysis in Health Care: Tools and Techniques, Third Edition

Tool Profile:
Cause-and-Effect Diagram (Synonyms: fishbone diagram, Ishikawa diagram)
(See Figure 7-5, page 155)

Stages to Use: Identifying proximate causes; identifying root causes

Purpose: To present a clear picture of the many causal relationships between outcomes and the contributing factors in those outcomes.

Simple Steps to Success:
1. Identify the outcome or problem statement.
2. Determine general categories for the causes.
3. List proximate causes under each general category.
4. List underlying causes related to each proximate cause.
5. Evaluate the diagram.

Tips for Effective Use
- Make sure everyone agrees on the problem statement or outcome.
- Be succinct and stay within the team's realm of control.
- Place the outcome on the right side of the page, halfway down, and then, from the left, draw an arrow horizontally across the page, pointing to the outcome.
- Represent common categories, including work methods, personnel, materials, and equipment, on the diagram by connecting them with diagonal lines branching off from the main horizontal line.
- Brainstorm to come up with the important proximate causes. Place each proximate cause on a horizontal line connected to the appropriate diagonal line.
- Gather data to determine the relative frequencies of the causes.
- Look for causes that appear continually in the evaluation process.
- Keep asking "Why?" to reach the root cause.
- Focus on system causes, not on causes associated with individual performance.

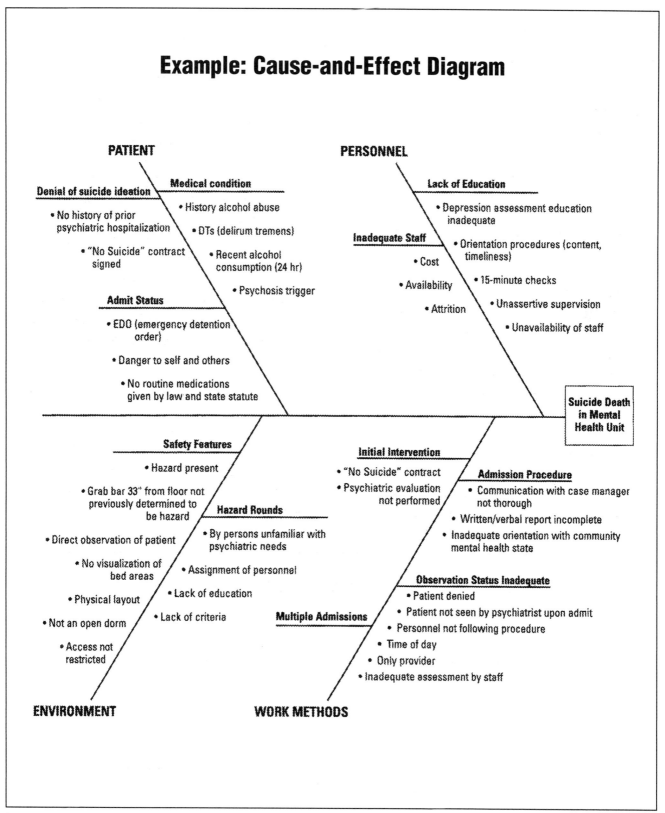

Figure 7-5. This figure illustrates how the generic diagram can be adapted to specific needs. This detailed diagram breaks down the contributing factors that led to a sentinel event—the suicide of a patient in a mental health unit. By analyzing the proximate and underlying causes listed, staff members can identify and prioritize areas for improvement.
Used with permission.

Tool Profile:
Change analysis
(See Figure 7-6, below)

Stages to Use: Identifying proximate causes; identifying root causes

Purpose: To determine the proximate and root cause(s) of an event by examining the effects of change. This involves identifying all changes, either perceived or observed, and all possible factors related to the changes.

Simple Steps to Success:
1. Identify the problem, situation, or sentinel event.
2. Describe an event-free or no-problem situation. Try to describe the situation without problems in as much detail as possible. Include the who, what, where, when, and how information listed in step 1.
3. Compare the two. Take a close look at the event and nonevent descriptions, and try to detect how these situations differ.
4. List all the differences.
5. Analyze the differences. Carefully assess the differences and identify possible underlying causes. Describe how these affected the event. Did each difference or change explain the result?
6. Integrate information and specify root cause(s). Identify the cause that, if eliminated, would have led to a nonevent situation.

Tips for Effective Use
- Describe the problem as accurately and in as much detail as possible. Include in the description who was involved, what was involved, where the event took place, when it took place, and what might have been a factor in causing the event.
- After a change analysis is performed, additional questions must be asked to determine how the changes were allowed to happen.
- Continue the questioning process into the organization's systems.
- Remember that not all changes create problems; rather, change can be viewed as a force that can either positively or negatively affect the way a system, process, or individual functions.

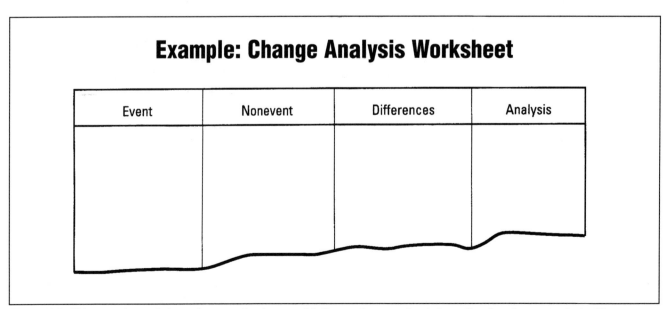

Figure 7-6. This generic worksheet shows a simple way of listing and comparing information for change analysis. The worksheet is arranged in columns to show logically what happened, what did not happen, the difference between them, and an analysis.

Tool Profile:
Control Chart
(See Figure 7-7, page 158)

Stages to Use: Identifying root causes; identifying opportunities for improvement; implementing and monitoring improvements

Purpose: To identify the type of variation in a process and whether the process is statistically in control.

Simple Steps to Success:
1. Choose a process to evaluate, and obtain a data set.
2. Calculate the average.
3. Calculate the standard deviation. The standard deviation is a measure of the data set's variability.
4. Set upper and lower control limits. Control limits should be three times higher or lower than the standard deviation relative to the mean.
5. Create the control chart. In creating the control chart, plot the mean (that is, centerline) and the upper and lower control limits.
6. Plot the data points for each point in time, and connect them with a line.
7. Analyze the chart and investigate findings.

Tips for Effective Use
- Obtain data before making any adjustments to the process.
- In plotting data points, keep the data in the same sequence in which they were collected.
- Be aware that special causes of variation must be eliminated before the process can be fundamentally improved and before the control chart can be used as a monitoring tool.
- Some special causes of variation are planned changes to improve the process. If the special cause is moving in the right direction toward improvement, retain the plan. It is working.
- The terms *in control* and *out of control* do not signify whether a process meets the desired level of performance. A process may be in control but consistently poor in terms of quality, and the reverse may be true.
- Charting something accomplishes nothing; it must be followed by investigation and appropriate action.
- Processes as a rule are not static. Any change can alter the process distribution and should trigger recalculation of control limits when the process change is permanently maintained and sustained (that is, greater than 8 to 12 points on one side of the process mean [centerline]).
- Four rules to identify out of control processes include the following:
  - One point on the chart is beyond three standard deviations of the mean
  - Two of three consecutive data points are on the same side of the mean and are beyond two standard deviations of the mean
  - Four of five consecutive data points are on the same side of the mean and are beyond one standard deviation of the mean
  - Eight data points are on one side of the mean

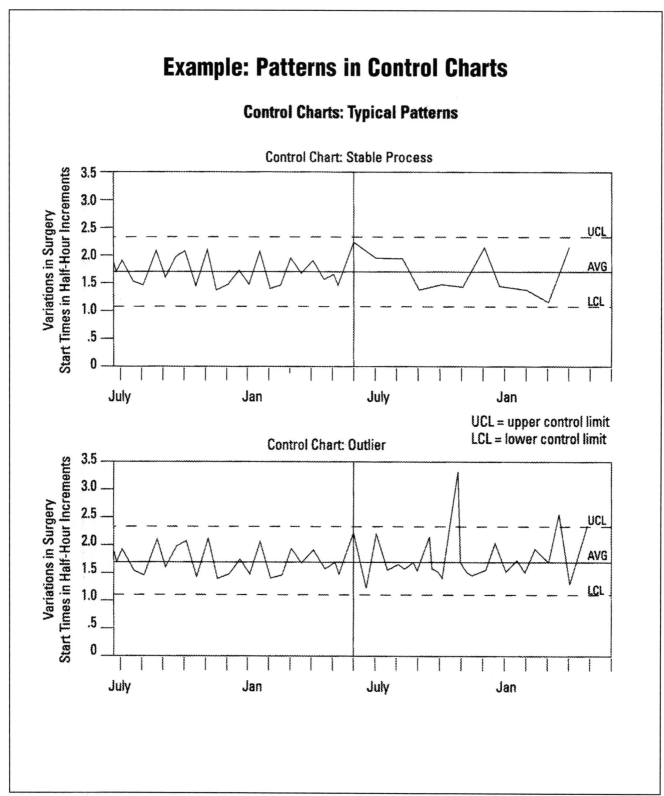

Figure 7-7. These two control charts illustrate different patterns of performance an organization is likely to encounter. When performance is said to be in control (top chart), it does not mean desirable; rather, it means a process is stable, not affected by special causes of variation (such as equipment failure). A process should be in control before it can be systematically improved. When one point jumps outside a control limit, it is said to be an outlier (bottom chart). Staff should determine whether this single occurrence is likely to recur.

Tools and Techniques **Chapter 7**

Tool Profile:
Failure mode and effects analysis (FMEA) (Synonym: failure mode, effects, and criticality analysis)
(See Figure 7-8, page 160)

Stage to Use: Identifying opportunities for improvement

Purpose: To examine a prospective design for possible ways in which failure can occur so that actions can be taken to eliminate the possibility of failure, stop a failure before it reaches people, or minimize the consequences of a failure.

Simple Steps to Success:
1. Select a high-risk process and assemble a team.
2. Diagram the process.
3. Brainstorm potential failure modes and determine their effects.
4. Prioritize failure modes (often accomplished through calculating a risk priority number).
5. Find root causes of failure modes.
6. Redesign the process.
7. Analyze and test the new process.
8. Implement and monitor the redesigned process.

Tips for Effective Use
- Risk priority numbers may be calculated as the product of ratings on frequency of occurrence, severity, and likelihood of detection.
- Remember that this type of analysis is generally proactive (used before an adverse event occurs), although use during root cause analyses to formulate and evaluate improvement actions is also recommended and described in this publication on page 110.

Example: Process for Failure Mode and Effects Analysis

① Item _____   ② Analysis Engineer _____
                                             Date _____
③ Function _____

Mode of Failure	Mechanism and Cause of Failure	Effects of Failure	Frequency of Occurrence	Degree of Severity	Chance of Direction
④	⑤	⑥	⑦	⑧	⑨

Risk Priority Number	Design Action	Design Validation
⑩ = ⑦ × ⑧ × ⑨	⑪	⑫

Failure Mode and Effects Analysis Form Entry Explanation

1. Item—Item to which analysis applies.
2. Analysis Engineer—An engineer in charge of design project.
3. Function—Function of the item as user perceives it. This description should be as broad as possible.
4. Mode of Failure—A mode in which the item will fail as perceived by user.
5. Mechanism and Cause of Failure—What causes failure to occur?
6. Effects of Failure—What effects will this failure have on the user or nearby person or nearby property?
7. Frequency of Occurrence (1–10)—How often is this failure expected to occur? This column is subjectively rated on a 1 to 10 basis.
   - 1 = Rare occurrence
   - 10 = Almost certain occurrence
8. Degree of Severity (1–10)—How severe is the effect of this failure on the user or anything else? This column is subjectively rated on a 1 to 10 basis.
   - 1 = Insignificant loss to user
   - 10 = Product inoperable or major replacement cost or safety hazard
9. Degree of Detection (1–10)—Can problem be detected by the user before it does the damage? This column is subjectively rated on a 1 to 10 basis.
   - 1 = Certain detection before failure
   - 10 = No detection possible before failure
10. Risk Priority Number (1–1,000)—Order of problem-solving priority is given by multiplying numbers in columns 7, 8, and 9.
11. Design Action—Action to reduce risk priority number.
12. Design Validation—Method to verify the design motion.

Figure 7-8. This chart shows a step-by-step process for performing FMEA. Joint Commission Resources' book titled *Failure Mode and Effects Analysis: Proactive Risk Reduction, Second Edition* provides detailed guidance on this proactive approach to risk reduction.

Source: Juran J.M., Gryna F.M.: *Juran's Quality Control Handbook, Fourth Edition*. New York: McGraw-Hill, Inc., 1988. Used with permission.

Tool Profile:
*Fault Tree Analysis
(Synonym: tree diagram)*
(See Figure 7-9, below)

Staged to Use: Identifying proximate causes; identifying root causes; identifying opportunities for improvement

Purpose: To provide a systematic method of prospectively examining a design or process for possible ways in which failure can occur, and to provide a graphic display of an event and the event's contributing factors.

Simple Steps to Success:
1. Define the top event of interest.
2. Construct the fault tree for the top event. List the major contributing factors under the top event as the first-level branches.
3. Continue the branching process by adding another level to the tree. These are the factors that might have accounted for the first-level branches.
4. Add additional levels of branching, as necessary.
5. Validate the tree diagram. Review the visualized events for accuracy and completeness.
6. Modify the diagram, as necessary. Retest the modified diagram.
7. Analyze the tree diagram. Identify possible problem scenarios.
8. Select the scenario that best fits the fact of the sentinel event or problem.
9. Determine the root cause of the event.
10. Recommend corrective and/or preventive actions.
11. Document the analysis and its results.

Tips for Effective Use
- Generally, the contributing factors can be grouped under such headings as personnel, material or equipment, procedures/processes, and so on.
- To validate the diagram, follow each of the paths through the tree for its fit with the facts of the sentinel event or accident. Is each factor plausible?
- Test and retest the tree diagram to "prune" the tree.
- The best-fit scenario is the scenario most likely to have resulted in the problem in terms of probability and/or the known facts of the particular situation.
- The root cause can be identified based on the inadequacies (causes) identified when listing possible scenarios.
- Corrective or preventive actions should be based on the event and root cause determination.

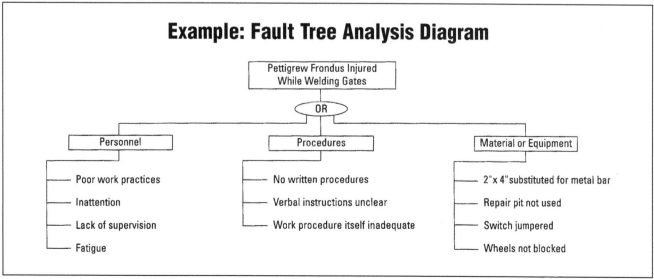

Figure 7-9. This diagram shows a fault tree constructed for a situation in which a maintenance worker was injured while making repairs. The first-level branches are divided into personnel, procedures, and material/equipment categories.
Source: Wilson P.F., Dell L.D., Anderson G.F.: *Root Cause Analysis: A Tool for Total Quality Management*. Milwaukee: ASQC Quality Press, 1993, p. 179. Used with permission.

Tool Profile: *Flowchart*
(See Figure 7-10, page 163)

Stages to Use: Identifying proximate causes; identifying root causes; identifying opportunities for improvement; implementing and monitoring improvements

Purpose: To help teams understand all steps in a process through the use of common, easily recognizable symbols; this illustrates the actual path a process takes or the ideal path it should follow.

Simple Steps to Success:
1. Define the process to be charted, and establish starting and ending points of the process.
2. Brainstorm activities and decision points in the process. Look for specific activities and decisions necessary to keep the process moving to its conclusion.
3. Determine the sequence of activities and decision points.
4. Use the information to create the flowchart. Place each activity in a box, and place each decision point in a diamond. Connect these with lines and arrows to indicate the flow of the process.
5. Analyze the flowchart. Look for unnecessary steps, redundancies, black holes, barriers, and any other difficulties.

Tips for Effective Use
- Ensure that the flowchart is constructed by the individuals actually performing the work being charted.
- Be sure to examine a process within a system, rather than the system itself.
- If the process seems daunting and confusing, create a simple high-level flowchart containing only the most basic components. Do not include too much detail; be wary of obscuring the basic process with too many minor components.
- Use adhesive notes placed on a wall to experiment with sequence until the appropriate one is determined.
- Make the chart the basis for designing an improved process, using spots where the process works well as models for improvement.
- Create a separate flowchart that represents the ideal path of the process, and then compare the two charts for discrepancies.
- Keep in mind that difficulties probably reflect confusion in the process being charted, and work through them.

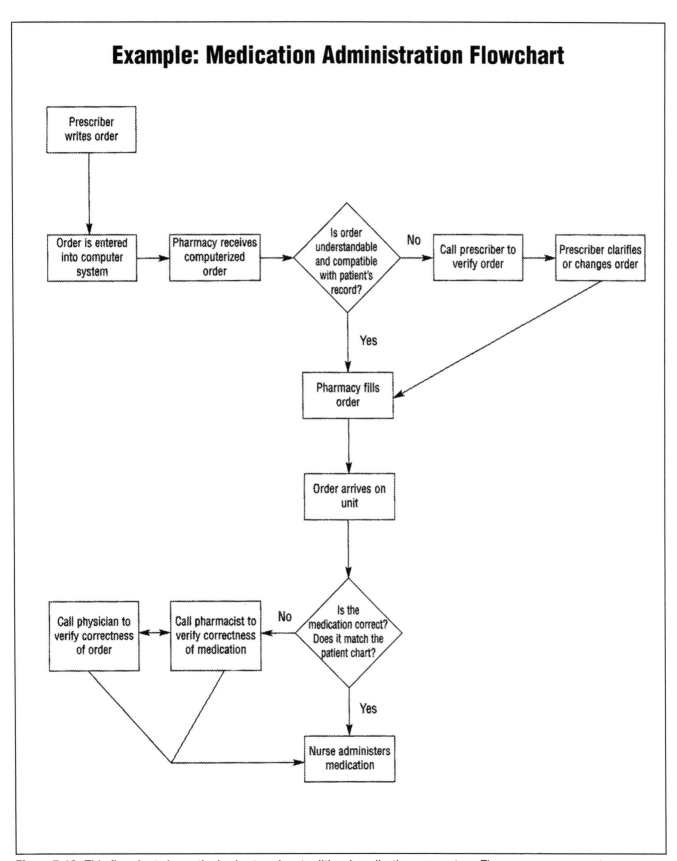

Figure 7-10. This flowchart shows the basic steps in a traditional medication-use system. The process components are arranged sequentially, and each stage can be expanded as necessary to show all possible steps.

Tool Profile:
Gantt chart
(See Figure 7-11, below)

Stages to Use: Identifying proximate causes; identifying root causes; identifying opportunities for improvement; implementing and monitoring improvements

Purpose: To graphically depict the timeline for long-term and complex projects, enabling a team to gauge its progress.

Simple Steps to Success:
1. Agree on start and stop dates for the project, and outline its major steps.
2. Draw a timeline.
3. Write the first step of the project under the appropriate time period. Enclose it in a rectangle long enough to stretch across the length of time estimated for completion.
4. Do the same for each of the succeeding steps.

Tips for Effective Use
- Leave enough space in the timeline to write beneath each time period.
- Write entries in a stair-step fashion, each step below the one before it, so that overlapping steps are clearly indicated.
- Color in the rectangles as each step is completed.
- If the project is very complex and lengthy, consider creating a Gantt chart for each phase or each quarter of the year.

Example: Gantt Chart

Task: Design Phase	Person(s) Responsible	Apr	May	Jun	Jul	Aug	Sep	Oct	Nov	Dec
Identify and appoint credentialing committee	SH	■								
Identify performance measures	SH and SR		■						■	■
Define policies and procedures that outline appointment, reappointment, and privileging process	SH and SR		■	■						
Develop credentialing application	SH and SR			■						

Figure 7-11. This Gantt chart of a competency and privileging process helped one team determine what tasks to undertake in what order. The chart details the target date and person(s) responsible for each task in the development process.

Tool Profile: *Histogram*
(See Figure 7-12, page 166)

Stages to Use: Identifying proximate causes; identifying root causes; identifying opportunities for improvement; implementing and monitoring improvements

Purpose: To provide a snapshot of the way data are distributed within a range of values and the amount of variation within a given process, suggesting where to focus improvement efforts.

Simple Steps to Success:
1. Obtain the data sets, and count the number of data points.
2. Determine the range for the entire data set.
3. Set the number of classes into which the data will be divided.
4. Determine the class width (by dividing the range by the number of classes).
5. Establish class boundaries.
6. Construct the histogram.
7. Count the data points in each class, and create the bars.
8. Analyze the findings.

Tips for Effective Use
- Data should be variable (that is, measured on a continuous scale such as temperature, time, weight, speed, and so forth).
- Make sure data are representative of typical and current conditions.
- Use more than 50 data points to ensure the emergence of meaningful patterns.
- Be sure that the classes are mutually exclusive so that each data point fits into only one class.
- Using K=10 class intervals makes for easier mental calculations.
- Be aware that the number of intervals can influence the pattern of the sample.
- To construct the histogram, place the values for the classes on the horizontal axis and the frequency on the vertical axis.
- Be suspicious of the accuracy of the data if the histogram suddenly stops at one point without some previous decline in the data.
- Remember that some processes are naturally skewed; do not expect a normal pattern every time.
- Large variability or skewed distribution may signal that the process requires further attention.
- Take time to think of alternative explanations for the patterns seen in the histogram.

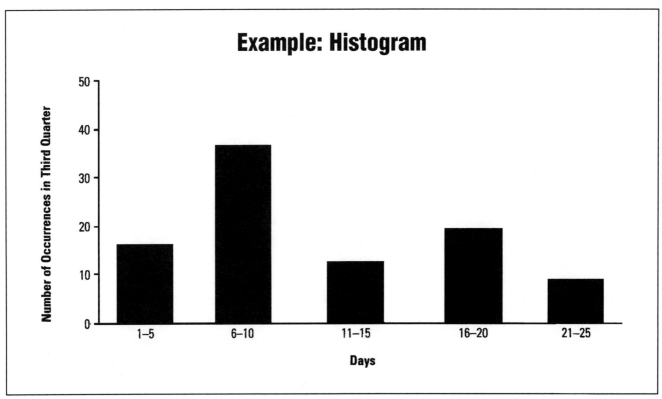

Figure 7-12. This sample histogram was developed by an infusion therapy service to analyze turnaround time for authenticating verbal orders from physicians. The irregular distribution suggests opportunities for improvement.

Tool Profile: *Multivoting*
(See Figure 7-13, below)

Stages to Use: Identifying proximate causes; identifying root causes; identifying opportunities for improvement

Purpose: To narrow down a broad list of ideas (that is, more than 10) to those that are most important and worthy of immediate attention. This involves reaching a team consensus about a list frequently generated by brainstorming.

Simple Steps to Success:
1. Combine any items on a brainstorming or other list that are the same or similar.
2. Assign letters to items on the new list.
3. Determine the number of points each group member can assign to the list. Each member uses a predetermined number of points (typically between 5 and 10) to vote on the different items on the list.
4. Allow time for group members to assign points independently.
5. Indicate each member's point allocation on the list.
6. Tally the votes.
7. Note items with the greatest number of points.
8. Choose the final group, or multivote again.

Tips for Effective Use
- Ensure that when combining ideas on the lists the team members who suggested the idea agree with the new wording.
- Use letters rather than numbers to identify each statement so that team members do not become confused by the voting process.
- Clearly define each idea so that it is easily understood by everyone voting.

Example: Multivoting

Improvement Opportunities	Number of Votes
A. Facility safety management	3
B. Patient education	7
C. Staff orientation	5
D. Referral (authorization)	3
E. Care coordination and communication	1
F. Laundry	7
G. Medication profile	5

Figure 7-13. This figure shows the results of multivoting on priorities for improvement at an Indian health center. The team was able to reach consensus on the need for prioritizing the laundering process.

Tool Profile: *Pareto chart*
(See Figure 7-14, page 169)

Stages to Use: Identifying root causes; identifying opportunities for improvement

Purpose: To show which events or causes are most frequent and therefore have the greatest effect. This enables a team to determine what problems to solve in what order.

Simple Steps to Success:
1. Decide on a topic of study. The topic can be any outcome for which a number of potential causes has been identified.
2. Select causes or conditions to be compared. Identify the factors that contribute to the outcome—the more specific the better.
3. Set the standard for comparison. In many cases, this is frequency, although factors may be compared based on their cost or quantity.
4. Collect data. Determine how often each factor occurs (or the cost or quantity of each, as appropriate). Use a check sheet to help with this task.
5. Make the comparison. Based on the data collected in the previous step, compare the factors and rank them from most to least.
6. Draw the chart's vertical axis. On the left side of the chart, draw a vertical line and mark the standard of measurement in increments.
7. List factors along the horizontal axis. Factors should be arranged in descending order, with the highest ranking factor at the far left.
8. Draw a bar for each factor. The bars represent how often each factor occurs, the cost of each factor, or its quantity, as applicable.
9. Include additional features, if desired. By making a few simple additions to the chart, a team can show the cumulative frequency, cost, or quantity of the categories in percentages.
10. Add up the percentages. All the percentage numbers for the causes need to add up to 100%.

Tips for Effective Use
- If the team is working from a cause-and-effect diagram, the topic is the effect that has been targeted for improvement.
- When selecting factors for comparison, beware of grouping several distinct problems together, which can skew the rank order. Refer to the cause-and-effect diagram, and use the most specific causes and factors possible.
- Be sure to mark the chart clearly to show the standard of measurement.
- When analyzing the chart, keep in mind that numbers do not always tell the whole story. Sometimes 2 severe complaints deserve more attention than 100 minor complaints.

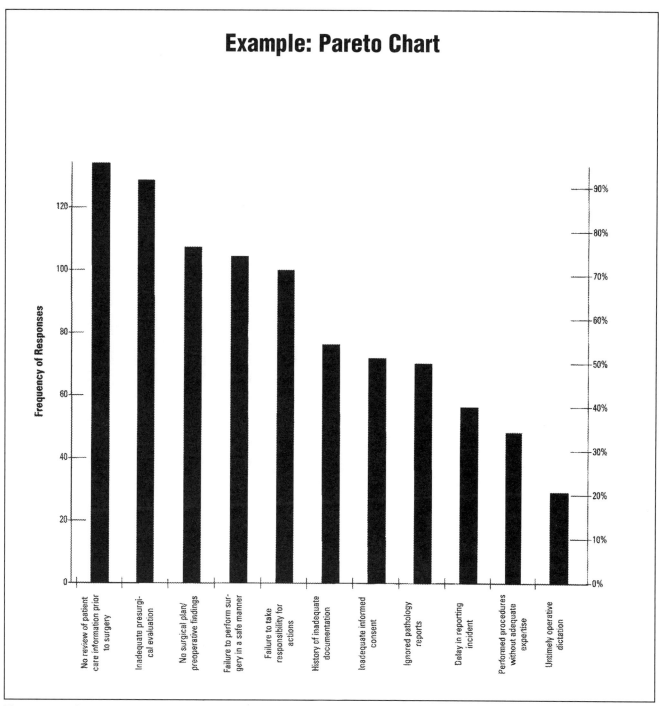

Figure 7-14. One organization used a Pareto chart to rank the frequency of responses of selected root causes provided by team members investigating a sentinel event involving a wrong-site surgery.
Used with permission.

Tool Profile: *Run Chart*
(See Figure 7-15, below)

Stages to Use: Identifying proximate causes; identifying root causes; implementing and monitoring improvements

Purpose: To identify trends and patterns in a process over a specific period of time so that teams can identify areas that require or are experiencing improvement.

Simple Steps to Success:
1. Decide what the chart will measure (what data will be collected over what period of time).
2. Draw the graph's axes.
3. Plot the data points, and connect them with a line.
4. Plot the centerline (that is, the overall average of all measurements).
5. Evaluate the chart to identify meaningful trends.
6. Investigate the findings.

Tips for Effective Use
- Make sure that the time period for data display is long enough to show a trend.
- Use at least enough data points to ensure detection of meaningful patterns or trends.
- Clearly mark all units of measurement on the chart. The x-axis should indicate time or sequence; the y-axis should indicate what is being studied.
- Indicate significant changes or events by drawing dashed lines through the chart at the appropriate points on the x-axis.
- Do not be too concerned with any one particular point on the chart (that is, wild points); instead, focus on vital changes in the process.
- Be aware that a run of six or more points on one side of the average indicates an important event or change.
- Integrate favorable changes into the system; take action to improve performance of unfavorable changes.

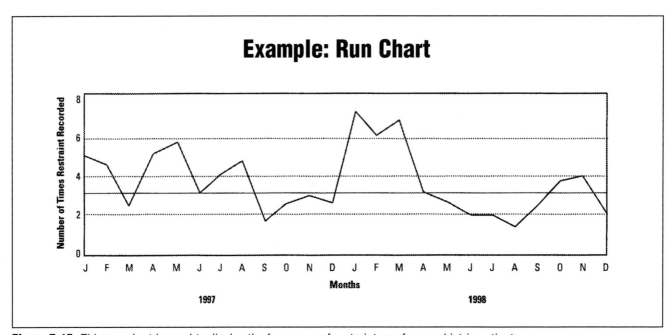

Figure 7-15. This run chart is used to display the frequency of restraint use for psychiatric patients.

Tool Profile:
Scatter Diagram
(Synonym: scattergram)
(See Figure 7-16, page 172)

Stages to Use: Identifying root causes; implementing and monitoring improvements

Purpose: To display the correlation—not necessarily the cause-and-effect relationship—between two variables.

Simple Steps to Success:
1. Decide which two variables to be tested.
2. Collect and record relevant data. Gather 50 to 100 paired samples of data involving each of the variables, and record them on a data sheet.
3. Draw the horizontal and vertical axes.
4. Plot the variables on the graph. If a value is repeated, circle that point as many times as necessary.
5. Interpret the completed diagram.

Tips for Effective Use
- Select two variables with a suspected relationship (for example, delays in processing tests and total volume of tests to be processed).
- Use the horizontal (x) axis for the variable you suspect is the cause and the vertical (y) axis for the effect.
- Construct the graph so that values increase while moving up and to the right of each axis.
- The more the clusters form a straight line (which could be diagonal), the stronger the relationship between the two variables.
- If points cluster in an area running from lower left to upper right, the two variables have a positive correlation. This means that an increase in y may depend on an increase in x; if you can control x, you have a good chance of controlling y.
- If points cluster from upper left to lower right, the variables have a negative correlation. This means that as x increases, y may decrease.
- If points are scattered all over the diagram, these variables may not have any correlation. (The effect, y, may be dependent on a variable other than x.)
- Remember, if the diagram indicates a relationship, it is not necessarily a cause-and-effect relationship.
- Be aware that even if the data do not appear to have a relationship, they may be related.
- Although scatter diagrams cannot prove a causal relationship between two variables, they can offer persuasive evidence.

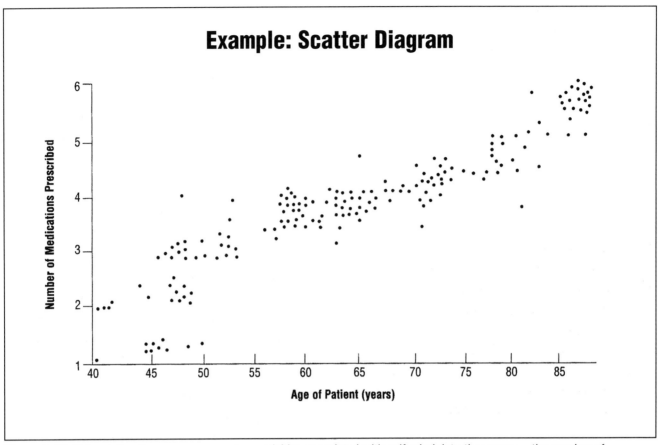

Figure 7-16. This scatter diagram compares two variables associated with self-administration errors—the number of medications prescribed and the ages of the patients involved. As might be expected, the clustering of points shows that the older the patient, the higher the number of medications involved in care.

Tool Profile: *Time Line*
(See Figure 7-17, below)

Stages to Use: Identifying proximate causes; identifying root causes

Purpose: To graphically display the temporal sequence of events.

Simple Steps to Success:
1. Draw a horizontal line across a piece of paper.
2. Establish time increments and note these on the horizontal line as vertical hatch marks.
3. Using arrows or vertical lines, note major events at the appropriate point along the timeline.
4. Using arrows or vertical lines, note major actions at the appropriate point along the timeline.

Tips for Effective Use
- Ask each key witness of an event to create a separate timeline. Compare these for patterns of agreement and disagreement.
- Separation of actions and events enhances the legibility of the timeline.
- You may wish to create a timeline of the ideal sequence of events and actions and then, to identify risk points and problems, compare this to the timeline of actual events and actions.

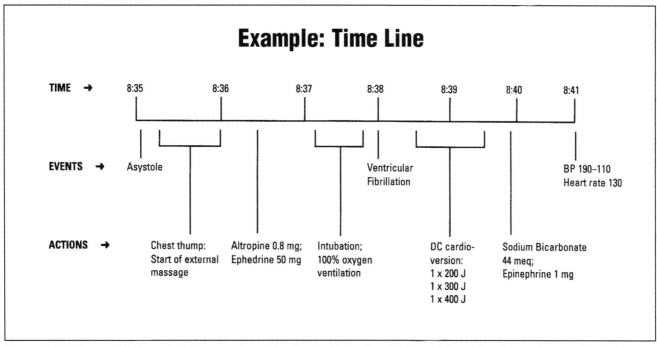

Figure 7-17. The graphic format of diagramming a timeline facilitates the display of information from a fast-moving incident. Readability is enhanced by the separation of actions and events. In this example, the time, events, and actions taken to handle an intraoperative cardiac arrest are displayed.
Source: Caplan R.A.: In-depth analysis of anesthetic mishaps: Tools and techniques. *Int Anesthesiol Clin* 27(3):157, 1989.

Chapter 8
Root Cause Analysis Case Studies

The following root cause analysis case studies were originally published in the January 2005 and March 2005 issues of the *Joint Commission Journal on Quality and Patient Safety*. This Joint Commission Resources publication is a monthly, peer-reviewed journal devoted to quality and patient safety.

The first root cause analysis case study, "Using Aggregate Root Cause Analysis to Reduce Falls and Related Injuries," focuses on an analysis of data from 176 root cause analyses of patient falls that occurred in the Department of Veterans Affairs (VA) system. This data was contributed by approximately 100 of the VA acute and long term care facilities. The case study discusses how the data was analyzed and how the organization measured the effectiveness of specific clinical changes at the bedside in reducing patient falls.

The second root cause analysis case study, "Learning to Improve Safety: False-Positive Pathology Report Results in Wrongful Surgery," examines a wrongful surgical resection; specifically, a radical retropubic prostatectomy that was performed on a 69-year-old male patient at the urology clinic at the Veterans Affairs Ann Arbor Healthcare System (VAAAHS) as a result of an erroneous pathology report. The case study investigates the events that contributed to the medical error and explains the recommendations of the root cause analysis team for new processes that were put in place as a result of the wrongful surgery. The case study also explains how compliance with the new policies was tracked.

Our sincere thanks go to these organizations for sharing their experiences with root cause analysis to assist colleagues at other organizations.

JOINT COMMISSION JOURNAL ON QUALITY AND PATIENT SAFETY

Root Cause Analysis

Using Aggregate Root Cause Analysis to Reduce Falls and Related Injuries

Peter D Mills, Ph.D., M.S.
Julia Neily, R.N., M.S., M.P.H.
Diana Luan, R.N., M.S.
Erik Stalhandske, M.P.P., M.H.S.A.
William B. Weeks, M.D., M.B.A., C.H.E.

Falls among the elderly are common, costly, dangerous, and often preventable. Approximately one-third of all adults 65 years of age and older are reported to fall each year. Persons living in institutions fall three times that rate (1.5 falls per bed per year), with as many as 25% of institutional falls resulting in fracture, laceration, or need for hospital care.[1-4] According to the Centers for Disease Control and Prevention, the cost of fall injuries for people ≥ 65 years of age is expected to reach $43.8 billion by 2020.[5] When compared to patients who had not fallen, patients with a hip fracture incurred increased health care costs of 78% to 101%.[6]

One method of determining the underlying causes of a fall is to conduct a root cause analysis (RCA).[7,8] Originally developed in high-hazard industries, RCA was mandated for investigation of all sentinel events in Joint Commission–accredited hospitals in 1997. In Department of Veterans Affairs (VA) hospitals, all serious adverse events and "potential" adverse events (near misses or close calls) are reviewed using RCA.[9] In certain categories of adverse events, such as falls and adverse medical events, in which there are many close calls, VA facilities may combine data from these events for a three- to six-month period and produce an aggregate review of the data in the category. Individual RCAs are still required for the more serious adverse events.

An aggregate review is an 11-step process (outlined in Figure 1 on page 22),[10] in which critical factors of the fall

Article-at-a-Glance

Background: In certain categories of adverse events, Department of Veterans Affairs (VA) facilities may combine data to produce an aggregate review of the data. Individual root cause analyses are still required for the more serious adverse events. About 100 of the VA acute and long term care facilities contributed data to an analysis of results of 176 root cause analyses (RCAs) for patient falls occurring in the VA system.

Methods: Success was measured through a decreased report of falls and major injuries due to falls after each organization's action plans were implemented. In addition, telephone interviews were conducted to understand success factors as well as barriers to implementation of clinical improvements.

Results: Of the 745 actions generated (that addressed the root cause), 435 (61.4%) had been fully implemented and another 148 (20.9%) had been partially implemented; 34.4% of the facilities reported reducing falls and 38.9% reported reducing major injuries due to falls.

Discussion: The action plans associated with these reductions focused on making specific clinical changes at the bedside rather than policy changes or educating staff. Specific interventions most highly associated with reductions in falls and injuries included environmental assessments, toileting interventions, and interventions that directly addressed the root cause and were the responsibility of a single person (as opposed to a group).

January 2005 Volume 31 Number 1

Overview of the Steps in the Aggregate Review Process

Step One
Charter Team
Gather and analyze data for specified time period

Step Two
Flow chart the general steps in the process

Step Three
Use text to describe how the team reviewed the general processes in the system

Step Four
Identify resources such as evidenced-based best practices, policies/procedures, and staff

Step Five
Determine the focus of this aggregate review

Step Six
Determine root cause/contributing factors; may use Triage/Triggering Questions and cause-and-effect diagram

Step Seven
Further develop root cause/contributing factors using the five rules of causation (NCPS Triage Cards)

Step Eight
Determine actions to address root causes

Step Nine
Write outcome measures for actions

Step Ten
Present analysis and actions to leadership for concurrence

Step Eleven
Implement actions and evaluate effectiveness; conduct aggregate root cause analyses on a regular basis

Figure 1. *An overview of the steps in the aggregate review process is shown.* Source: VA National Center for Patient Safety. *Triage/Triggering Questions:* Concept Definitions for Triggering and Triage Questions.™ http://www.patientsafety.gov/concepts.html (last accessed Oct. 26, 2004); Cause-and-effect diagram: Root Cause Analysis Tools *(internal document).* Ann Arbor, MI, Version: August 2002; Using the Five Rules of Causation: http://www.patientsafety.gov/causation.html (last accessed Oct. 26, 2004); NCPS Triage Cards: Concept Definitions for Triggering and Triage Questions.™

(for example, time, location, medications, environmental conditions) are analyzed together for all of the falls occurring in a specific time period. On the basis of this analysis, common root causes are determined and actions are developed to ameliorate them. The advantage of the aggregate review is that the actions taken to improve care are based on data from multiple events and therefore have the potential to address problems common to many falls.

Preventing Falls

Several strategies have been determined to be effective in reducing falls. Each begins with an accurate assessment of the patient's fall risk, followed by interventions such as exercise programs, including balance and gait training and strengthening exercise, evaluation of postural hypotension, and medication review with modifications to reduce falls. Patient education (again, as part of a multifactorial program) is also important in fall reduction. Consideration should be given to the assessment and treatment of osteoporosis to decrease the risk of fractures.[11,12] Assistive devices (such as bed alarms, canes and walkers, hip protectors) may be helpful as part of a multifactorial intervention program.[11]

Although strategies for reducing falls are known, implementation is a challenge. It is also difficult to determine if the same approaches that reduce falls will also reduce injuries due to falls.[12] Our research on reducing falls and related injuries suggest that the most effective interventions for reducing major injuries due to falls are the following:[13]

- Toileting interventions
- Use of signage to identify high-risk patients
- Use of hip-pads
- Environmental interventions
- Staff education
- Postfall assessments

Once root causes and prevention strategies are identified, the difficult work of implementation begins. Grol and Grimshaw[14] outlined the following basic issues affecting clinician change:

- Attributes of the change
- Barriers to making a change
- Implementation strategy

Journal ON QUALITY AND PATIENT SAFETY

Changes that are compatible with existing values and skills, supported by good evidence, and less complex, and that require fewer organizational changes are more likely to be adopted. In addition, Rogers found "relative advantage to be one of the best predictors of an innovation's rate of adoption."[15(p.216)] Barriers to change can occur at the individual level (for example, beliefs about the change or its effects), team level (for example, prevailing practice, habits of opinion leaders), and organizational level (such as lack of time and resources, effective systems of communication).[16] Finally, the implementation strategy must be tailored to the type of change being made. Generally, passive dissemination of educational material is less effective, and active, collaborative, and multifaceted interventions are more likely to work.[17]

The VA National Center for Patient Safety was interested in the primary causes of falls in the VA system and the primary means by which facilities were attempting to reduce falls. Further, we wanted to understand which interventions implemented to reduce falls and injuries due to falls were the most effective as well as what tools or facility characteristics aided in the implementation of these interventions. To examine these questions, the research team (J.N., K.H.H.) analyzed the aggregate RCA reports for falls in the VA system and interviewed staff that submitted these analyses.

We examined the following hypotheses:
- Sites that implemented actions that represented concrete changes in care delivery (as opposed to changes in policy or recommendations for more staff education and training) would be the most successful at reducing fall and major injury rate
- Sites that had participated in the falls collaborative (an eight-month Collaborative Breakthrough Series on reducing falls and injuries due to falls in the VA system, which was conducted between July 2001 and March 2002 with 37 VA and non-VA teams[13]) would be more successful in implementing interventions and reducing falls and fall related injuries than sites that had not participated in the falls collaborative
- Sites would report minimal reductions in fall rates and modest reductions in major injury rates; we found similar results in the falls collaborative project (described above)

Methods

This descriptive study examined 176 aggregate fall RCAs completed at 97 of the 173 Veterans Health Administration (VHA) acute and long term care facilities. We read and coded 176 aggregate fall RCAs submitted from October 1999 to June 2002. We phoned each site to ask about the implementation of actions and success factors for implementation. We coded the aggregated RCAs using an instrument that achieved an 89.5% agreement between the coders.

Structured Interview

All 97 facilities that submitted at least one aggregate review were called and interviewed by the research team. The patient safety manager or designee at each facility was interviewed by a research team member using a structured interview. The goal of the interviews was to determine whether facilities were able to implement the action plans produced as a result of their aggregate RCA and whether those actions had led to reported reductions in falls and injuries due to falls. For each proposed action, we asked if it had been fully or partially implemented, whether the facility had reduced falls and injuries due to falls, whether they were not measuring these variables, or whether it was "too soon to tell" if reduction had occurred.

We also inquired about success factors and barriers to improvement perceived by the patient safety managers as well as specific tools that, if provided, would help them in their work. When asking about success factors and barriers to improvement, we inquired about a list of common factors and then asked about any other factors the interviewee believed to have helped or hindered the implementation. These questions were dichotomously scored "yes" or "no."

Analysis

We used descriptive statistics to report the numbers and types of root causes identified, the action plans developed, and the primary success factors and barriers to implementation of action plans identified by the patient safety managers. We computed the rate for implementation of actions for each facility by dividing the number of actions fully implemented by the total number of actions. For example, if a facility planned 20 actions and completed 10 of them, the implementation rate would be .5. The implementation rate provided a marker of the facilities' ability to implement actions, which is a prerequisite for successful improvement. Spearman's Rho nonparametric correlations were used to analyze the relationship between rates of implementation and barriers to change. We also analyzed the relationship between specific action plans that were implemented and reported reductions in falls or major injuries using nonparametric correlational analysis (Phi Coefficient for 2×2 tables).

Results

Ninety-seven facilities completed 176 aggregate RCAs that aggregated 10,701 specific patient falls. These RCAs uncovered 478 root causes, which resulted in 745 actions to address the root causes. The RCAs averaged 63.32 cases aggregated per report (standard deviation [SD] = 52.63), 2.8 root causes (SD = 1.94), and 4.46 actions (SD = 3.30) and took an average of 47.80 person hours each (SD = 32.40).

Root Causes

The root causes found for falls and injuries related to falls involved problems with polices or procedures (44%), communication problems (23%), the need for more training (16%), environmental causes (13%), and fatigue or scheduling problems (4%). Figure 2 (page 25) displays the specific categories for the reported root causes. The "staff needs more training" category represented more than 16% of the reported root causes, followed by the need for specific interventions for specific patient populations (14.4%), and the need to improve the current system for falls assessment (14.2%). Other common categories were as follows:
- Need to improve documentation of falls (7.7%)
- Improved communication of fall risk (7.5%)
- Need for specific equipment (5.6%)
- No system to assess fall risk (5.4%)

Implementing Action Plans

We analyzed each action plan to see whether it addressed the intended root cause and found that 95% (708) of the 745 actions did in fact address the root cause. Of those actions that addressed the root cause, 435 (61%) were reported to be fully implemented and another 148 (21%) were partially implemented. Staff or patient education involved 27.2% of the actions, 40.4% of the actions involved changes or improvements in policy, and 32.4% involved specific changes in patient care (Table 1 on page 26). We asked the patient safety managers, "Which actions had the most impact on reducing falls and injuries due to falls?" The Appendix displays the responses for facilities reporting clinical improvement.

For the 202 action plans that involved education, 172 (84.93%) involved staff education and 20 (9.93%) involved patient education. For the 301 action plans involving policy change, 48 (15.84%) focused on changing policies regarding prefall assessment tools, 39 (13.12%) focused on other (unspecified) tools to improve falls documentation, and 31 (10.40%) focused on general policy to improve falls assessment. For the 241 action plans that focused on making specific clinical changes, 48 (20.06%) focused on deploying assistive devices to reduce falls or injuries due to falls, 29 (12.04%) focused on improving signage to identify high-risk fallers, and 26 (10.8%) focused on making environmental interventions (see Table 1 on page 26).

Overall Reduction in Falls and Injuries Due to Falls

A reduction of falls was reported by 34.4% of patient safety managers, 43.8% of patient safety managers reported no change, and 20.8% reported that it was too soon to tell. In addition, 38.9% of patient safety managers reported reducing major injuries, 26.3% reported no change, and 31.6% reported that it was too soon to tell. Note that only 1% of the facilities were not measuring their rate of falls and that only 3.2% were not measuring their major injuries.

Facilitators and Barriers

Figure 3 (page 27) displays behaviors that the patient safety managers reported helped facilitate implementation of their action plans and the primary barriers. Figure 4 (page 28) displays the resources that patient safety managers found to be the most helpful, and Figure 5 (page 28) displays a list of resources that would be helpful in reducing falls and related injuries.

Facilities that reported using the same team to implement change (that was used to conduct the root cause analyses) had higher implementation rates (Rho = .226,

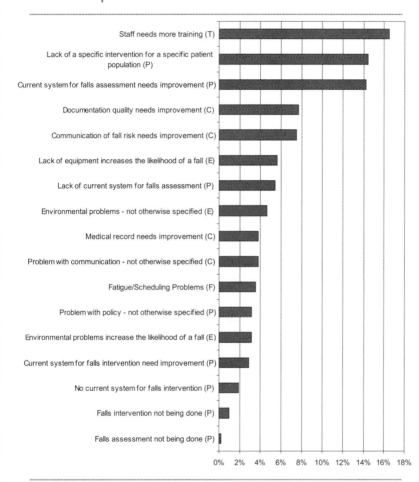

Figure 2. *Percentages for specific root causes of falls are shown. T, Training; P, Policy/Procedures; C, Communication; E, Environmental; F, Fatigue/Scheduling.*

$p = .04$). The following three barriers were associated with a lower implementation rate:
- Not using the same team to implement changes (Rho = –.292, $p = .011$)
- Not getting feedback from the staff before attempting to implement change (Rho = –.248, $p = .023$)
- Not enough time or resources to implement the actions (Rho = –.278, $p = .009$)

It is important to note that a facility's overall rate of implementation was not associated with decreases in major injuries (Rho = –.078, $p = .449$) or falls (Rho = –.068, $p = .508$), so reports of implementation alone may not be a good measure of improved clinical outcomes.

When examining correlations between the implementation of an action plan and reductions in falls and injuries due to falls, we found that environmental assessments (Phi = .121, $p = .012$), toileting interventions (Phi = .124, $p = .010$), actions that specified making clinical changes (Phi = .165, $p = .001$), and identification of a specific individual responsible for carrying out the action plan (Phi = .093, $p = .054$) were associated with a reduction in falls. Toileting interventions (Phi = .124, $p = .033$) and actions that specified making clinical changes (Phi = .145, $p = .003$) were associated with reductions in major injuries. Actions that specified staff education were negatively correlated with reports of decreased falls (Phi = –.144, $p = .003$) or major injuries (Phi = –.130, $p = .007$).

Finally, 18 of the 97 teams we interviewed had participated in a Collaborative Breakthrough Series on reducing falls and injuries due to falls that took place from July 2001 to March 2002. This participation was significantly correlated with reported reductions in falls (Phi = .217, $p = .03$) and major injuries from falls (Phi = .335, $p = .001$).

Discussion

This is the first study that has analyzed a series of RCAs of aggregated data on patient falls, the responses of the

Table 1. Action Plan Categories for Falls Aggregate RCAs

Category of Action	Percentage of Total	Percentage of Category	Category of Action	Percentage of Total	Percentage of Category
Education and Training	**27.20%**		**Making Clinical Changes**	**32.40%**	
Staff education and training (any program that educates staff)	23.10%	84.93%	Assistive devices (not otherwise specified)	6.50%	20.06%
Patient education and training (any program that educates patients)	2.70%	9.93%	Nonslip footwear	0.10%	0.31%
Education and training - not otherwise specified	1.40%	5.15%	Special walkers	0.30%	0.93%
Policy Change	**40.40%**		Alarms	1.50%	4.63%
Tools and templates to improve falls documentation (not otherwise specified)	5.30%	13.12%	Hip protectors	0.80%	2.47%
Specifically prefall risk assessment tool	6.40%	15.84%	Signage (may include wristbands, signs on doors, falling stars, anything that identifies the patient at risk)	3.90%	12.04%
Specifically postfall assessment tool	1.80%	4.46%	Environmental assessment and intervention (may include special high risk for fall rooms, or a room designated for high risk patients, or environmental rounds, i.e., floor waxing)	3.50%	10.80%
Policy about assessment or an assessment tool	4.20%	10.40%	Toileting interventions	2.30%	7.10%
Improvement of incident report documentation	3.50%	8.66%	Use of interdisciplinary team	1.50%	4.63%
Interdisciplinary team	1.50%	3.71%	Performing postfall assessment	1.20%	3.70%
Medications review (seeks to reduce the risk of falls due to medications)	1.10%	2.72%	Exercise program (any type of exercise program such as physical therapy, Tai Chi, strengthening)	1.10%	3.40%
Toileting intervention	0.80%	1.98%	Verbal actions to improve communication of risk (i.e., shift to shift, discipline to discipline)	1.10%	3.40%
Exercise program (any type of exercise program such as physical therapy, Tai Chi, strengthening)	0.10%	0.25%	Medications review (action that seeks to reduce the risk of falls due to medication)	0.80%	2.47%
Policy change - not otherwise specified	15.70%	38.86%	**Clinical changes - not otherwise specified**	7.80%	24.07%

system to those root causes, and their outcomes across multiple settings. We found that 82% of actions were at least partially implemented as a result of an RCA, resulting in 34.4% of facilities reporting reduced falls and 38.9% reporting reduced major injuries due to falls. The action plans associated with these reductions were plans that focused on making specific clinical changes at the bedside rather than making policy changes or educating staff. In fact, we were surprised to find that action plans that specified staff education were actually negatively correlated with reports of reduced falls and major injuries. Specific interventions that were most highly associated with reductions in falls and injuries included environmental assessments, toileting interventions, and interventions that directly addressed the root cause and that were the responsibility of a single person (as opposed to a group).

Categories of Root Causes and Actions

Both the most common general category of root cause—"the need to improve a policy or procedure," including the lack of specific interventions for a particular patient population and the need to improve systems for assessment of risk—and the second-most common root cause—"the need to improve the communication of risk"—can lead to specific changes in the system that will enhance clinical care. Even though the need for staff training (the third most popular category of root causes and the single most popular specific type of root cause) can be a legitimate root cause, it can also be a simplistic solution to a complex problem. For example, if initial falls assessments are not being done, one reason may be that the staff is not adequately trained, but other reasons could include lack of time, staffing shortages, or other organizational issues.

We have several recommendations regarding training. First, make sure that a skills deficit actually exits when designating the need for training as a root cause, especially when the training aims to improve the skills that staff would be expected to have already (as opposed to training in conjunction with new procedures or equipment). Second, look for other, systemic, reasons why

Joint Commission Journal on Quality and Patient Safety

Helpful Behaviors and Barriers in Implementing Action Plans

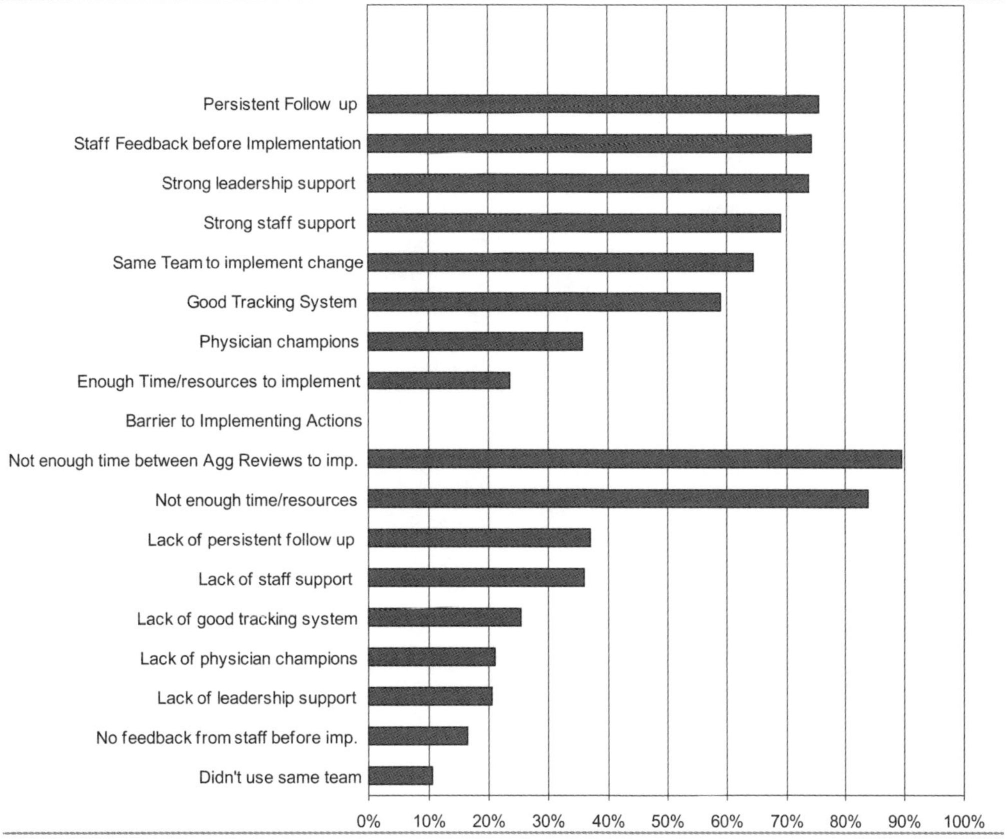

Figure 3. *Percentages of patient safety managers endorsing the helpful behaviors and barriers in implementing action plans are shown.*

staff was not able to perform a specific task, such as fatigue, distraction, time pressure, or other competing clinical duties. Third, be sure to measure not only whether the staff received training but also changes in staff behaviors and patient outcomes, such as reduced falls and related injuries that are expected to result from the training intervention.

In examining the superordinate categories of actions, we found that only those actions representing specific clinical changes were associated with reductions in falls and major injuries. Although policy changes may be needed, it should not be assumed that they will lead to improvements in clinical outcomes. In fact, it may be more effective to conduct a trial of a new clinical change, refine the process, and then solidify the change with a policy.

Facilitators and Barriers to Change

In our interviews, we were able to identify facilitators and barriers to change. More than 70% of the patient safety managers reported that persistent follow-up, staff feedback before implementation, and strong leadership support were helpful to implementation. This finding is consistent with our previous analysis[18] of 143 medical improvement teams, in which we found that support from front-line staff and leadership were characteristic of high-performing teams. Our finding that facilities which used the same team to implement the action plan and to

Helpful Resources in Implementing Action Plans

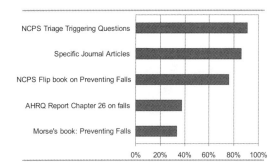

Figure 4. *The percentages of patient safety managers who found the listed resources as helpful are shown. Helpful resources for implementing an action plan include the Veterans Affairs National Council for Patient Safety (NCPS) Triage Triggering Questions, a flipbook of 78 questions designed to help identify the root cause of a medical incident; the* Flip Book on Preventing Falls, *a book of specific interventions designed to reduce falls and injuries due to falls (http://www.patientsafety.gov; Chapter 26 of the AHRQ Report (Agostini, J.V., Baker, D.I., Bogarus, Jr., S.T.: Prevention of falls in hospitalized and institutionalized older people. In:* Making Health Care Safer: A Critical Analysis of Patient Safety Practices. *Rockville, MD: Agency for Healthcare Research and Quality, 2001, pp. 281–299); and Morse J.M.:* Preventing Patient Falls. *Thousand Oaks, CA: Sage Publications, 1997.*

conduct the RCA were more likely to implement the change is also consistent with our analysis of the 143 teams, in which we found that a team which had worked together before were more likely to be high performers.

The most commonly reported barrier to implementing actions was limited time since the last falls aggregate review. When we conducted the interviews, the patient safety managers in the VA system conducted an aggregate review of falls data every three months. Some of the action plans were not yet fully implemented by the time the next aggregate review was conducted. We have addressed this issue by increasing the period between reports to six months.

The second most commonly reported barrier to implementation was the lack of time and resources, which suggests that senior leaders should be concerned that identified risks may not be addressed because of lack of resources. The negative correlation between failure to get feedback from the front-line staff before implementing and the rate of implementation suggests the need to test changes before implementation. One model for testing change is the Plan-Do-Study-Act cycles of change,[19] which was part of our curriculum for the Collaborative Breakthrough Series on reducing falls and related injuries—in which participation was correlated with improved clinical outcomes.

The tools that facilities used to identify the root causes and to develop and implement action plans (Figures 4 and 5), including the triage-triggering questions and flipbook on preventing falls, are available on the VA National Center for Patient Safety Web site.[20] On the basis of these results, we have developed a "Falls Tool Kit" to be available on the Web.

Resources that Would Help Implement Action Plans

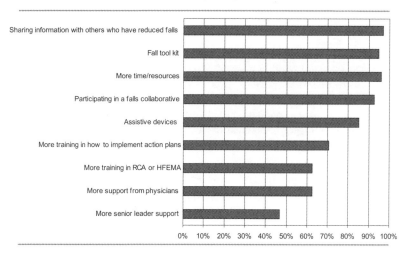

Figure 5. *A list of resources that would be helpful in reducing falls and related injuries is shown. RCA, root cause analysis; HFMEA, Healthcare Failure Mode and Effects Analysis™.*

Identifying the Most Effective Interventions

Even though this was not a treatment outcome study, we were interested in identifying interventions that were associated with the greatest clinical change. We found that actions which focused on clinical change were highly correlated with reports of reduced falls and injuries due to falls. Within this category of actions, we also found that conducting environmental assessments and implementing toileting interventions were also independently associated with improved outcomes. This finding replicates the results of the Collaborative Breakthrough Series on reducing falls, in which we also found that environmental assessments and toileting interventions, implemented in the context of a multifactorial program, reduced major injuries.[13]

Our finding that it is better to have a single identified person responsible for carrying out actions rather than a group—so as not to diffuse responsibility—has led us to promote this strategy in our work with improvement teams. In addition, having found that implementation alone was not related to improved clinical outcomes, we do not recommend using the number of actions "implemented" as a measure of positive change. Rather, facilities should report changes in clinical outcomes, such as falls or injuries due to falls, as markers of improvement.

Limitations

This study has several limitations. First, our results are based solely on the written and verbal reports of the patient safety managers at the local facilities and therefore are associative and not causative. Second, we did not independently verify the process by which root causes were identified or action plans developed; nor did we verify the patient safety manager's reports of actions implemented or reductions in falls or injuries. Third, it is difficult to determine which actions were responsible for reductions in falls or injuries because all the facilities implemented several actions simultaneously, and the success of a specific action results from a complex combination of patient, facility, and staff characteristics that work together to produce positive clinical change. Facilities may also have been implementing interventions to reduce falls before implementing their aggregated review action plans. Finally, the magnitude of associations, while statistically significant, is relatively small, indicating that the majority of variance in falls and major injuries remains unexplained.

Conclusions

Despite these limitations, this analysis of aggregate patient fall RCAs points to several main results. First, actions that result in direct clinical changes at the bedside are more effective than changes in policy or staff education. Second, using the RCA teams to implement changes, giving a single individual responsibility for implementing actions, getting feedback from staff before implementing the change, and giving the team the time and resources needed will all increase the chances of implementing an action plan. Third, using implementation alone is not a conclusive measure of improved clinical outcomes; rather, it is important to measure actual changes in clinical outcomes. Fourth, participation in the Collaborative Breakthrough Series on reducing falls appears to have helped facilities reduce falls and injuries due to falls and taught them the skills to continue to do so over the long run.

This article is the result of work supported with resources and the use of facilities at the Veterans Affairs National Center for Patient Safety in Ann Arbor, Michigan, and the Veterans Affairs Medical and Regional Office Center, White River Junction, Vermont. The local Internal Review Board (IRB) approved this project.

Peter D. Mills Ph.D., M.S., is Associate Director, Field Office, VA National Center for Patient Safety, White River Junction, Vermont. **Julia Neily, R.N., M.S., M.P.H.,** is Nurse Associate Director and **Diana Luan R.N., M.S.,** is Health Science Specialist, Field Office, VA National Center for Patient Safety, White River Junction, Vermont. **Erik Stalhandske, M.P.P., M.H.S.A.,** is Program Manager, VA National Center for Patient Safety, Ann Arbor, Michigan. **William B. Weeks, M.D., M.B.A., C.H.E.,** is Director, Field Office, VA National Center for Patient Safety, White River Junction, Vermont. Please address reprints requests to Peter Mills, Ph.D., Peter.Mills@med.VA.gov.

References

1. Rubenstein L., Josephson K.R., Robbins A.S.: Falls in the nursing home. *Ann Intern Med* 121:442–451, Sep. 15, 1994.
2. Doweiko D.: Prevention program cut patient falls by 10%. *Hosp Case Manag* 8:38, 43–44, Mar. 2000.
3. Rubenstein L., Powers C.M., MacLean C.H.: Quality indicators for the management and prevention of falls and mobility problems in vulnerable elders. *Ann Intern Med* 135:686–693, Oct. 16, 2001.
4. Hoskin A.F.: Fatal falls: Trends and characteristics. *Stat Bull Metrop Insur Co* 79:10–15, Apr.–Jun. 1998.
5. Centers for Disease Control and Prevention: *A Toolkit to Prevent Senior Falls: The Costs of Fall Injuries Among Older Adults.* National Center for Injury Prevention and Control. http://www.cdc.gov/ncipc/factsheets/fallcost.htm (last accessed Oct. 21, 2004).
6. Brainsky A., et al.: The economic cost of hip fractures in community-dwelling older adults: A prospective study. *J Am Geriatr Soc* 45:281–287, Mar. 1997.
7. Joint Commission on Accreditation of Healthcare Organizations: *2003 Comprehensive Accreditation Manual for Hospitals: The Official Handbook.* Oakbrook Terrace, IL: Joint Commission on Accreditation of Healthcare Organizations, 2002.
8. Wald, H., Shojania K.G.: Root cause analysis. In: *Making Health Care Safer: A Critical Analysis of Patient Safety Practices.* Agency for Healthcare Research and Quality, 2001, pp. 51–56.
9. Bagian, J.P., et al.: Developing and deploying a patient safety program in a large health care system: You can't fix what you don't know about. *Jt Comm J Qual Improv* 27:522–532, Oct. 2001.
10. Neily J., et al.: Using aggregate root cause analysis to improve patient safety. *Jt Comm J Qual Improv* 29:434–439, Aug. 2003.
11. American Geriatrics Society, British Geriatrics Society, and American Academy of Orthopaedic Surgeons Panel on Falls Prevention: Guideline for the prevention of falls in older persons. *J Am Geriatr Soc* 49:664–672, May 2001.
12. Tinetti, M.E : Clinical practice: Preventing falls in elderly persons. *N Engl J Med* 348:42–49, Jan. 2, 2003.
13. Mills P.D., et al.: Reducing falls and fall-related injuries in the VA system. *J Healthcare Safety* 1:25–33, 2003.
14. Grol R., Grimshaw J.: From best evidence to best practice: Effective implementation of change in patients' care. *Lancet* 362:1225–1230, Oct. 11, 2003.
15. Rogers, E.M.: *Diffusion of Innovations, 4th Ed.* New York: The Free Press, 1995, pp. 216.
16. Cabana M., et al.: Why don't physicians follow clinical practice guidelines: A framework for improvement. *JAMA* 282: 1458–1465, Oct. 20, 1999.
17. Grimshaw J.M., et al.: Changing physicians' behavior: What works and thoughts on getting more things to work. *J Contin Educ Health Prof* 22:237–243, Fall 2002.
18. Mills, P.D., Weeks W.B.: Characteristics of successful quality improvement teams: Lessons from five collaborative projects in the VA. *Jt Comm J Qual Saf* 30:152–162, Mar. 2004.
19. Langley G.J., et al.: *The Improvement Guide: A Practical Approach to Enhancing Organizational Performance.* San Francisco, Jossey-Bass, 1996.
20. Department of Veterans Affairs: VA National Center for Patient Safety. http://www.patientsafety.gov (last accessed Oct. 21, 2004).

Appendix. Actions Identified by Patient Safety Managers as "Having the Biggest Impact on Reducing Falls and Injuries due to Falls"*

- Revise our initial assessment measure from invalidated measure to one (Morse fall scale[†]) that is becoming the standard for the VA.
- Admission nurse continues to send e-mail to unit ID team to identify patient at risk for falls and initiate interim fall care plan. Night nurse will review fall interventions on care plan and will respond on the email the fall prevention strategies already in place and make any further recommendations and then update the care plan accordingly. Provide education on new process.
- Identify one nursing unit that will participate in a pilot using yellow dots to identify patients at high fall risk.
- Establish a fall workgroup to review the fall prevention program policy draft focusing on the fall risk assessment and reassessment process to include the following objectives:
  1. Simplify the overall process.
  2. Explore use of other validated/reliable assessment tools such as the Morse fall scale.
  3. Evaluate the feasibility of using one assessment tool for one area and another for acute care and psychiatry.
  4. Computer linkage of the electronic fall risk assessment and the new admission assessment template.
  5. Automatic scoring of the fall risk assessment template.
  6. Delete the initial 24-hour monitor at admission.
  7. Eliminate the moderate risk designation.
  8. Define triggers for reassessment.
  9. Delete all previous fall supplemental review forms.

Appendix. Actions Identified by Patient Safety Managers as "Having the Biggest Impact on Reducing Falls and Injuries due to Falls," *continued*

- Facilitywide educational blitz and follow-up reinforcement education plan for Fall Risk Program, including identifiers.
- The Morse fall risk assessment tool will be used to assess patients for risk of falling.
- Establish process of offering toileting to patients at risk for falling every two hours to prevent anticipated physiological falls.
- The fall prevention pyramid will be implemented on 9N. All nursing staff and treatment team members of 9N will receive an in-service on this model.
- Review and revise guidelines for repeat falls.
- Continue to focus on reducing the severity of injuries related to falls by using hipsters, low beds, and the Morse fall assessment tool.
- Ensure communication regarding patient at risk for falling. Post fall risk in the alert/warning section of the computerized medical record cover page of patient designated as high risk for falling.
- A staff member is to be specifically assigned to conduct fall prevention rounds as per the facility policies on each team-oriented unit, ensuring that the rounds are completed by 12/15/01.
- Develop patient incident reporting tool for falls through computerized medical record, incorporating data elements related to fall risk assessment, fall prevention plan, and postfall evaluation.
- Reinforce facilitywide use of the fall prevention program as outline in nursing service memo #2.
- Procurement of brake extensions and bright colored tennis type balls needs to occur. A systematic procedure needs to be developed so that these items are appropriately installed on wheelchairs in current use. Routine ward supply of these items needs to be available for use when stock or new chairs are issued for use by residents on unit. The trial of new safety devices such as automatic locking brakes with a frequent faller to test efficacy of product needs to occur.
- Design and implement a hospital wheelchair program that includes maintenance and inventory/replacement.
- Assessment of each unit's need for additional collapsible walkers (collapsible for easier storage). The team already assessed specific units.
- Enhance staff awareness of the increase risk for fractures when four-sided rails are used.
- Prepare and distribute patient education pamphlet on wheelchair safety for patient and staff use.
- Develop a laminated card that includes reminders about wheelchair safety and attach to wheelchair.
- Recommend trial use of rubber lined/fluid absorbing rugs in patient rooms by bedside.
- Need assessment for fall potential to include more than Morse fall scale.

* ID, Identification; ICU, intensive care unit.

† Morse J.M.: *Preventing Patient Falls*. Thousand Oaks, CA: Sage Publications, 1997.

Joint Commission Journal on Quality and Patient Safety

Root Cause Analysis

Learning to Improve Safety:
False-Positive Pathology Report Results in Wrongful Surgery

Marcia M. Piotrowski, R.N., M.S.
Roland L. Bessette, J.D.
Stephen Chensue, M.D., Ph.D.
Daniel Cutler
Allen Kachalia, M.D., J.D.
James W. Roseborough
Sanjay Saint, M.D., M.P.H.
Willie Underwood III, M.D., M.S., M.P.H.
Hedwig S. Murphy, M.D., Ph.D.

Mr. "Jonathan Kilpatrick," a 69-year-old patient, was referred by his primary care physician to the urology clinic at the Veterans Affairs Ann Arbor Healthcare System (VAAAHS). The purpose of the referral was to evaluate the patient's mildly elevated prostate specific antigen (PSA) level of 4.58 ng/mL. The physician had palpated a nodule on the right side of the prostate gland and recommended that Mr. Kilpatrick have a biopsy to rule out malignancy.

In December 2002 the patient underwent a transrectal ultrasonography and prostate biopsy. No abnormalities were found on the sonograph. A total of 10 cores of prostatic tissue were taken with a biopsy needle. The surgical pathology report stated: "Prostate, right and left lobes, biopsies; positive for prostatic adenocarcinoma, Gleason grade 3 + 4 for a total score of 7 involving both sides, approximately 34% of the specimen submitted. Perineural invasion not identified." Of note, the pathologist was not provided with the patient's PSA level at the time of diagnosis.

Two weeks after the biopsy the patient was seen in the urology clinic. The physician explained the risks, benefits, and complications of both surgical and nonsurgical treatment options. Mr. Kilpatrick elected surgery. In February 2003 he underwent a radical retropubic prostatectomy with bilateral pelvic lymph node dissection. The pathologist found that the specimen from the surgical resection was negative for prostate adenocarcinoma. The earlier biopsy slides were rereviewed and no definitive adenocarcinoma

Article-at-a-Glance

Background: A patient experienced a wrongful surgical resection, specifically, a radical retropubic prostatectomy because of a false-positive pathology report.

Findings from the Root Cause Analysis (RCA): The RCA team identified three antecedent events that contributed to this medical error: (1) a second (concurring) pathologist did not provide a written opinion, (2) a single pathologist who reviewed and signed the final report, and (3) a pathologist who did not review the case and reconfirm the diagnosis immediately prior to the surgical resection.

Recommendations: The RCA team recommended that the concurring pathologist write his or her diagnostic findings on the referral form, two pathologists review and sign the final typed report, and a pathologist rereview the slides on the business day prior to a surgical resection. Because the prostate specific antigen (PSA) value can be helpful in select cases of prostate cancer, the team recommended the PSA value be referenced when reviewing prostate specimens obtained through fine-needle biopsy.

Tracking Compliance: Because a wrongful surgical resection is a rare event, emphasis was placed on measuring compliance with distinct elements that were part of the revised procedure. During a 12-month span, practitioners demonstrated sustained compliance to the enhanced process for analyzing and reporting results.

was identified. The chief of the pathology and laboratory medicine service, together with other pathologists, performed an extensive review of all prostate biopsies performed over a several-day period before, during, and after the time of the errant biopsy report to determine if the original slides for Mr. Kilpatrick had been incorrectly labeled and belonged to a different patient. No evidence of mislabeling was found.

"To err is human. To forgive is not the policy of this hospital." This message hung in a room used for new employee orientation nearly three decades ago. Although it captured attention it likely did little to prevent medical error. When a mistake occurs there is a strong cultural norm to apportion punishment to individual practitioners.[1-2] There is also an incentive to affix blame because this is a gateway to compensation through the tort system.[3] However, medical safety experts emphasize that imposing professional sanctions is not the most productive approach to error reduction. Instead, systems should be created that will both reduce the probability of untoward events and make mistakes visible when they do occur, thereby capturing errors before they reach patients.[4-10]

Because patient safety is a vital component of health care quality, the Joint Commission for Accreditation of Healthcare Organizations mandates the conduct of a thorough and credible root cause analysis (RCA) for those errors resulting in either patient death or significant patient morbidity. A well-done RCA focuses on process and system factors and will ideally result in the implementation of risk-reduction strategies.[11]*

In contrast to the health care industry, where individual medical centers conduct RCAs, the National Transportation Safety Board (NTSB), established in 1967, "conducts independent investigations of all civil aviation accidents in the United States and major accidents in the other modes of transportation." Addressing safety deficiencies is a vital function of the NTSB. To promote change as quickly as possible, the board often releases safety recommendations before the investigation is complete.[12] Detailed information on each accident is readily available to the public. For example, an Air Midwest flight crashed in Charlotte, North Carolina, on January 8, 2003, killing 2 crew members and 19 passengers.[13] Both the cause of and factors contributing to the crash are listed in the executive summary released by the NTSB.[14] Safety recommendations are addressed to the Federal Aviation Administration, with the intent of improving safety across the entire airline industry.[15]

This article provides the results of the RCA performed following the case of wrongful surgical resection, as described at the outset, because of a false-positive pathology report at VAAAHS in Ann Arbor, Michigan. A Midwestern medical center, VAAAHS is a teaching and comprehensive research facility with 4 campuses, a close affiliation with a major medical school, and affiliations with more than 40 other health care organizations.

Case-based learning is a long-established educational tool, allowing an in-depth presentation of clinical complexities.[16-17] Sharing an actual scenario sparks far greater clinician interest than simply describing a generic safety deficit.[18] Remedial actions in response to Mr. Kilpatrick's case were designed to create a more robust procedure for reviewing and releasing pathology reports. The solutions had to be both achievable and feasible within the resources of the pathology and laboratory medicine service. Because an unnecessary surgical resection cannot be reversed, the safety net had to be extremely strong to prevent the mistake from reaching the patient. No single antecedent resulted in the untoward event.[1] Rather, a combination of situational factors converged, abetted by procedural weaknesses and resulting in a misdiagnosis of adenocarcinoma.

Conducting the RCA

To understand the weaknesses that contributed to the wrongful surgery it is important to subdivide the system for managing pathology specimens into three phases:
- In the *preanalytic* phase, specimens are obtained from the patient and transported to the pathology section.
- The *analytic* phase commences with the arrival of specimens at the pathology receiving station and terminates with the release of the pathology report.
- The *postanalytic* phase involves the receipt and follow-up of the pathology report by the ordering clinician.

Table 1 (page 125) lists each step in the analytic procedure and the phase during which this error occurred.

---

* Standard PI.2.30, "Processes for identifying and managing sentinel events are defined and implemented." [PI-11]

Journal on Quality and Patient Safety

Table 1. Handling Pathology Specimens During Analytic Phase

#	Step in Procedure
1	Deliver biopsy specimens, accompanied by requisition form, to pathology receiving
2	Information on requisition form is matched with specimens received
3	Resident physician in pathology records number of specimens and number of tissue cores received
4	Process specimens
5	Prepare slides
6	Deliver slides and requisition form to primary pathologist
7	Primary pathologist ensures that number of slides received matches number of specimens recorded on requisition form
8	Primary pathologist makes preliminary diagnosis and may dictate a report
	If slides represent an initial diagnosis of malignancy or if pathologist desires second opinion, then slides reviewed by second, or concurring, pathologist
9	Deliver slides to concurring pathologist
10	Concurring pathologist provides agreement or conflicting opinion
	Findings handwritten on requisition form
11	If primary and consulting pathologists do not reach diagnostic concensus, obtain third opinion from consulting pathologist
12	Primary pathologist dictates final report
13	Secretary transcribes final report
14	Concurring pathologist reviews final report
15	*Concurring pathologist reviews and signs final report*
	Primary pathologist reviews, signs, and releases final report
16	*Pathologist rereviews slides on business day before patient scheduled for definitive surgical resection*

* Procedural steps added folowing root cause analysis.

Sequence of Events

The clinical risk manager [M.M.P.] interviewed key clinicians—the primary pathologist, concurring pathologist, resident physician in pathology, and chief of the pathology and laboratory medicine service. The error, unknown at the time, occurred when the pathologic diagnosis was made following the prostate biopsy. Discovery of this error occurred nine weeks after the prostatectomy was performed. The lapse of time resulted in suboptimal recollection of details by physicians involved with this case. Although the exact nature of the miscommunication could not be established, the following description represents the most likely sequence of events. Mr. Kilpatrick's preliminary diagnosis, given by the primary pathologist, was adenocarcinoma of the prostate. Because this case represented a first diagnosis of malignancy the slides were sent to a second, or concurring, pathologist within the pathology department for review. The second pathologist saw no evidence of adenocarcinoma. At the time this error occurred, it was not customary practice for the concurring pathologist to document his or her findings in writing. It was likely that the resident physician transported the slides between these two staff physicians, although the chain of custody was not recorded. It is uncertain whether the concurring pathologist's findings were verbally communicated directly between the two staff pathologists or through an intermediary (that is, the resident physician). The final diagnostic report, indicating adenocarcinoma, was dictated by the primary pathologist and transcribed by the secretary. At the time of the untoward event, the typed names of both the primary and concurring pathologist were on the final report, but only one pathologist reviewed, signed, and released the report, after which there were no further steps to allow recovery from the error.

Procedural Weaknesses

An RCA team's task is to thoroughly explore an adverse incident until both the immediate (proximate) and underlying (root) causes have been identified. With the aid of a flowchart depicting the chronological sequence of events, the incident was discussed at length. Although an error in pathology always involves a particular type of specimen, the team recognized that many of its findings should be widely applicable to all pathology specimens, regardless of the tissue type. This in-depth review resulted in the construction of a cause-and-effect diagram (Figure 1, page 126). The dissemination of a false-positive pathology report was the proximate cause of the event. However, the lack of a safe and effective communication process in diagnostic pathology was the system failure and the root cause of the error.

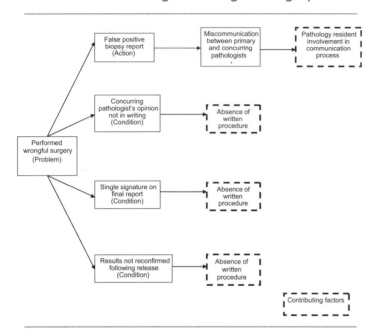

Figure 1. *The RCA team constructed a flowchart to depict the incident.*

Exploring further, the RCA team identified two specific weaknesses in written communication that directly contributed to the untoward outcome, which were as follows:
- The concurring pathologist was not required to put his or her opinion in writing.
- The names of both the primary and concurring pathologists were on the final diagnostic report, but only one pathologist was required to review and sign the report before release.

The RCA team identified an additional deficit, wherein a neoplastic diagnosis was not reconfirmed just before a therapeutic surgical resection. Even in the presence of suboptimal communication, a terminal review of the pathology slides had the potential to prevent the error from reaching the patient.

Associated Issues

Although the RCA team primarily focused on procedural weaknesses, members also requested information on other skill-based issues that could potentially contribute to the risk of error. The team asked for a presentation on difficulties associated with the diagnosis of prostate adenocarcinoma and an explanation of how pathologist competency is maintained. The team was also interested in the response to the error—when and how the mistake was disclosed to Mr. Kilpatrick and his family.

A pathologist [H.S.M.] informed the RCA team about several issues consistently raised regarding prostate biopsy diagnoses. Interobserver variability,[19] difficulties in interpretation of atypical foci,[20-21] and atypia in non-neoplastic prostate glands after hormonal or radiotherapy[22] are traditional pitfalls in prostate diagnosis. More recently, several studies have recommended the cutpoint for biopsy be lowered to 2.5 ng/mL for all men aged 60 years and younger.[23-24] These changes in interpretation of clinical laboratory values have led to biopsy of patients with relatively lower PSAs, resulting in the increasing incidence of prostate biopsies with the presence of very small foci of adenocarcinoma or atypical glands and subsequent prostatectomy specimens with low-volume cancer. Further complicating this area is a study that shows when a biopsy was prompted by an elevated PSA level obtained before surgery, in many cases the PSA level returned to less than 4 ng/mL before surgery.[25] The increasing number of cases in which minute foci of carcinoma are identified has increased interest in the development of a number of immune markers that are helpful in confirming diagnoses made on histopathology and are now used routinely at the VAAAHS. Recognizing these challenges helped the team understand why there had been a difference in clinical opinion between the primary and concurring pathologists when diagnosing Mr. Kilpatrick's specimens.

The RCA team explored maintenance of practitioner competencies. The surgical pathologists in the department are board certified in anatomic pathology.

Pathologists maintain their competency via a number of informal and formal venues and are regularly evaluated by both internal and external review programs. Pathologists independently attend national conferences, which include specialized courses in surgical pathology. An in-house lecture series, "Topics in Pathology," brings in outside pathologists with subspecialty expertise to discuss relevant topics in diagnostic surgical pathology. In addition, because all pathologists are faculty members of the pathology department in a highly affiliated, university-based health care system, they have access to all lectures and presentations within that department. Quarterly, the Armed Forces Institute of Pathology (AFIP) issues four to five cases with clinical history and glass slides to VAAAHS pathologists, who return their diagnoses to the AFIP. In turn each pathologist receives an expert review of the case. All pathologists at the VAAAHS consistently score well on the AFIP reviews. Finally, within the department, a second pathologist reviews a 10% sample of all cases in a timely manner. Discrepancies are noted and addressed. This intensive, multilayered system for ensuring individual practitioner competency convinced the RCA team that the error was likely a result of procedural weaknesses and not due solely to deficits in the skill level of the individual pathologists involved.

The clinical risk manager told the team that disclosure of the error had been accomplished promptly, before the RCA was conducted. Initially the surgeon revealed the adverse event during a clinic visit arranged with the patient and his family. Two family meetings followed. Attendees included the patient and his wife and children, the urologic surgeon [W.U.], the chief of the pathology and laboratory medicine service [S.C.], and the clinical risk manager [M.M.P.]. In the final meeting, which was conducted after the RCA was completed, the resulting action plan was communicated. Ample time was allowed for questions. Through these formal interactions the patient came to appreciate the honesty of the clinicians. He told us that he would likely have never known of the error without our honesty. Following these meetings, the patient decided to submit a Claim for Damage, Injury, or Death, a standard form prescribed by the Department of Justice and used by the Department of Veterans Affairs. A legal settlement was achieved.

Recommendations

The RCA team's goal was to identify actions with broad applicability. With only one exception, the recommendations were intended to improve the analytic procedure for all pathology specimens not just prostate biopsies. Steps to enhance the procedure, summarized in Table 1 (page 125), are outlined below.

First, the concurring pathologist should write his or her opinion on the requisition form. This second opinion would be obtained before release of the final report. This would help ensure accurate communication between the primary and concurring pathologists. The recommendation does not preclude a discussion between the two physicians but supported this discussion with written confirmation of findings.

Second, it had been an established practice to send select cases to a consulting pathologist who was not employed at the VAAAHS. Although the failure to use an outside consultant did not contribute to this particular error, the team felt it was an integral component of the analytic phase of diagnostic pathology and should be addressed. Consultative opinions were obtained for difficult diagnoses, particularly in cases in which the primary and concurring pathologists could not reach consensus. Most consultants were from a local university-based health care system. The procedure for obtaining the consultant's opinion had not been highly structured. To assist in monitoring compliance it was recommended that the procedure become more formalized.

Third, the concurring pathologist would review and sign the final typed diagnostic report. The signature of the primary pathologist would continue to be a requirement. Written confirmation by two pathologists would protect the patient from an erroneous diagnosis by ensuring dual agreement with the report prior to release.

Fourth, on the business day preceding each surgical resection a pathologist would rereview the patient's biopsy slides to confirm the diagnosis. The repeat review would be analogous to a final quality check before shipping a manufactured product.

The final recommendation—that the pathologist reference the patient's PSA value before determining the histopathologic diagnosis—was supplementary to the other recommendations. In select cases, this action can serve as a trigger for careful rereview of the specimen.

Table 2. Re-review of Diagnostic Pathology Specimens Prior to Surgical Resection*

Date	Patient	Social Security Number	Case Number	Reviewing Pathologist (Initials)	Comments
4/1/04	A	–	04-8574	RT	Squamo-basal cell ca to margins
4/2/04	B	–	03-7389	RT	Lymphoma
4/2/04	C	–	04-5521	GS	Breast cancer
4/5/04	D	–	04-3493	JW	Negative biopsy; clinical decision to perform resection
4/6/04	E	–	04-1823	RT	Prostate ADC
4/6/04	F	–	03-8534	LS	Skin cancers; multiple
4/8/04	G	–	03-7942	LS	SCCA; cytology and biopsy
4/9/04	H	–	04-3733	GS	Melanoma in situ
4/12/04	I	–	04-9836	KE	ADC of colon

*Information has been changed to protect confidentiality of patients and pathologists; ca, cancer; ADC, adenocarcinoma; SCCA, squamous cell cancer.

For example, if the pathologist diagnoses extensive high-grade adenocarcinoma of the prostate, but the PSA is normal, the diagnosis and identifying information would be reexamined for possible error. The RCA team recommended that the urologist performing the prostate biopsy should record the PSA value on the pathology requisition form. If the urologist failed to enter this information, the primary pathologist would attempt to electronically access the PSA value before determining a diagnosis.

Tracking Compliance with Recommendations

Wrongful surgery secondary to a diagnostic error in pathology is a rare event. Although it is appropriate to track the frequency with which similar errors occur, it is important to augment that data with other measures. The RCA team devised methods for assessing compliance with the revised procedures within the pathology service.

Pathologists maintained a comprehensive tracking form for patients whose slides were rereviewed on the day before a surgical resection (Table 2, above). Each month the clinical risk manager abstracted five cases involving organ resection from the surgery service schedule. The number of surgical resections performed on the basis of an abnormal preoperative pathology report ranged from 7 to 17 cases per month, with a mean of 13 cases. Therefore, this monthly sample was at least 29% and as high as 71% of the total cases. These names were cross-matched to the tracking form to ensure that patients were not being missed. Data were collected for nine months and reported to our medical center's performance improvement committee. Seven percent (3) of the cases were not documented on the tracking form. In retrospect we found that one of these cases had been reviewed but inadvertently not recorded on the tracking form. Another case had not been reviewed because the type of surgery (for example, below the knee amputation) was usually not dependent upon an abnormal preoperative pathology report. Only one case had been missed without an explanation. Because there was a consistently high level of compliance with the procedure the frequency of the monitor was reduced. Spot checks are now conducted two months during each year.

On a monthly basis, documentation from 100% of the internal and external pathology consultations was retrospectively reviewed to ensure each consult was appropriately completed and signed by the reviewing pathologist. The number of external consultations ranged from 13 to 37, with a mean of 24.33 consultations per month. As part of this effort a form was created to simplify data collection and guide extra-departmental consultants (Table 3, page 129). During a one-year period compliance improved substantially (Figure 2, page 130), from 78% to 100%. Although a high level of compliance is being maintained, this is such a critical procedure that monthly monitoring continues.

Completed pathology reports were reviewed each month to make certain both the primary and concurring physicians had signed. For the first 6 months following the

Table 3. Reporting Form for Pathology Consultations Sent to Other Agencies

VA Ann Arbor Healthcare System (VAAAHS)
Interdepartmental Consultation Report Form

VAAAHS Accession Number (year must be included) _____

Surgical Pathology (SP) _____

Cytology (CY) _____

Consultant's Opinion

_____
_____
_____

This opinion applies to whole case   Yes _____   No _____
If no, then this applies only to parts _____
_____

Signature _____
Date _____

---

change to a more robust procedure requiring two signatures, 100% of the reports were reviewed for the presence of both signatures, with the number of monthly reports for internal or external consultations ranging from 50 to 85, with a mean of 67 reports. Since then a 10% sample of reports have been reviewed. Data reflecting compliance is reported to our hospital's Invasive Procedure Committee. For 9 of the first 12 months (March 2003–February 2004) following implementation of the RCA team's recommendations, compliance was 100%, with compliance at 97% for 1 month and 95% for 2 of the months.

Disseminating Information

Promoting patient safety is a cherished value of VAAAHS. The goal is accomplished through a variety of activities. When a major event occurs, such as this error, it is widely shared across the organization. A one-page sheet, "Lessons Learned," summarizes the adverse event, core messages, and actions taken (Figure 3, page 130). The form, designed in close collaboration with our medical illustrator, is simple and uncluttered. Key points are bulleted and an illustration provides visual appeal. The purpose of the "Lessons Learned" is to stimulate discussion that will lead to a greater understanding of patient safety and the spread of change.

Unfortunately, the lessons learned from an RCA are rarely disseminated beyond the institution conducting an in-depth analysis. The reasons for this cultural censorship[26] include the following:

- Negative public perception of the institution
- Vulnerability to legal liability*
- Possible accreditation issues
- Embarrassment and shame for the involved clinicians[6,27-31] Paradoxically, this hesitancy to publicly disclose errors—to bring mistakes out of the shadows—prevents transference of learning. It is deceptively difficult to craft solutions to safety problems.[32] Working in a vacuum, without building on the experience of others, increases the challenge and the risk.

Conclusions

"Experience and common sense both tell us that when well-intentioned, skilled individuals independently use the same complex rules to solve a problem, their final conclusions often are different."[33(p. 1)] In a review of surgical pathology in a university hospital, 1.2% of surgical reports contained important errors, which could have affected patient management. Despite recognition of the sources of these errors, this percentage remained constant in the

---

* It can be argued that liability as a result of court action exerts pressures for systemic improvement. However, the assessment of such liability on a case-by-case basis creates a conflict wherein medical institutions and practitioners must isolate occurrences with a potential for liability and assume a defensive posture. Thus, the benefits that could be realized from an open forum are thwarted.

Journal on Quality and Patient Safety

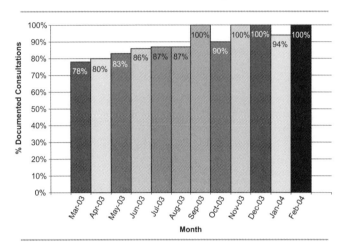

Figure 2. *All consultations are reviewed monthly to measure the percentage appropriately completed and signed by the consulting pathologist.*

Figure 3. *A one-page sheet, "Lessons Learned," summarizes the adverse event, core messages, and actions taken.*

ensuing years.[23-24] Although errors may have a variety of origins, certainly one of the most difficult dilemmas faced by pathologists is that which arises from diagnostic variation (a term describing the situations in which, given the same surgical specimen, pathologists may arrive at differing interpretations). Even among experts in subspecialty areas of diagnostic surgical pathology, independently reviewing cases, there is variability in final diagnoses to the extent that clinical outcomes for patients would be substantially and significantly different.[34-36] Some diagnostic interpretations are exceedingly and notoriously difficult, and often errors are identified only after recognition of inconsistency between the original diagnosis and the clinical outcome.[37] Some persons feel that given the complex nature of medical practice, the multitude of clinical data, and the interventions that each patient receives, a high error rate is perhaps not surprising.[38]

In the adverse event described here, the difference in diagnoses between the two pathologists was not unexpected. An independent dual diagnosis of the same specimen was a sound process that decreased the risk of error by allowing two opinions. The difficulty was a failure to discuss and resolve that diagnostic variability. This lack of discussion and resolution of the diagnosis resulted from weaknesses in the communication process that had not been recognized until this untoward event occurred. Developing safer systems is an incremental and ongoing process requiring sustained vigilance. Sharing lessons learned promotes learning both within and outside organizational boundaries. **J**

Dr. Saint is supported by a Career Development Award from the Health Services Research & Development Program of the Department of Veterans Affairs and a Patient Safety Developmental Center Grant from the Agency for Healthcare Research and Quality (P20-HS11540).

March 2005 Volume 31 Number 3

Joint Commission Journal on Quality and Patient Safety

Marcia M. Piotrowski, R.N., M.S., formerly Clinical Risk Manager, VA Ann Arbor Healthcare System (VAAAHS), Ann Arbor, Michigan, is Infection Control Coordinator, and a member of the *Joint Commission Journal on Quality and Patient Safety*'s Editorial Advisory Board. **Roland L. Bessette, J.D.,** is Regional Counsel, Department of Veterans Affairs, Detroit. **Stephen Chensue, M.D., Ph.D.,** is Chief, Laboratory and Pathology Medicine Service, VAAAHS. **Daniel Cutler** is a Medical Illustrator, VAAAHS. **Allen Kachalia, M.D., J.D.,** formerly Chief Medical Resident, Department of Internal Medicine, University of Michigan Medical School, Ann Arbor, is Attending Hospitalist, Department of Medicine, Brigham and Women's Hospital, Boston. **James W. Roseborough** is Director, VAAAHS. **Sanjay Saint, M.D., M.P.H.,** is Research Investigator, VA Center for Practice Management and Outcomes Research, VAAAHS. **Willie Underwood III, M.S., M.D.,** is Chief, Urology Service/Department of Surgery, VA Center for Practice Management and Outcomes Research. **Hedwig S. Murphy, M.D., Ph.D.,** is Pathologist, Laboratory and Pathology Medicine Service, VAAAHS. Please address reprint requests to Marcia M. Piotrowski, R.N., M.S., Marcia.Piotrowski@med.va.gov.

References

1. Grasha A.F.: Into the abyss: Seven principles for identifying the causes of and preventing human error in complex systems. *Am J Health-Syst Pharm* 57:554–564, Mar. 15, 2000.
2. Wu A.W.: Medical error: The second victim (editorial). *BMJ* 7237:727–728, Mar. 18, 2000.
3. Runciman W.B., et al.: Error, blame, and the law in health care: An antipodean perspective. *Ann Intern Med* 138:974–979,E-980, Jun. 17, 2003.
4. Moray N.: Error reduction as a systems problem. In Bogner M.S. (ed.): *Human Error in Medicine.* Hillsdale, NJ: Erlbaum, 1994, pp. 67–91.
5. Institute of Medicine: *To Err Is Human: Building a Safer Health System.* Washington, D.C.: National Academy Press, 2000.
6. Berwick D.M.: Taking action to improve safety: How to increase the odds of success. *Proceedings of Enhancing Patient Safety and Reducing Errors in Health Care,* Nov. 8–10, 1998. Chicago: National Patient Safety Foundation, American Medical Association, 1999, pp. 1–10.
7. Reason J.: Human error: Models and management. *BMJ* 7237:768–770, Mar. 18, 2000.
8. Nolan T.W.: System changes to improve patient safety. *BMJ* 7237:771–773, Mar. 18, 2000.
9. Leape L.L.: Foreword: Preventing medical accidents: Is "systems analysis" the answer? *Am J Law Med* 27(2-3):145–148, 2001.
10. Buerhaus P.I.: Lucian Leape on the causes and prevention of errors and adverse events in health care: Interview by Peter I. Buerhaus. *Image J Nurs Sch* 31(3):281–286, 1999.
11. Joint Commission on Accreditation of Healthcare Organizations: *2004 Comprehensive Accreditation Manual for Hospitals: The Official Handbook.* Oakbrook Terrace, IL: Joint Commission Resources, 2004.
12. National Transportation Safety Board: *About the NTSB: The Investigative Process.* http://www.ntsb.gov/abt_ntsb/invest.htm (last accessed Jan. 11, 2004).
13. News & events: *Air Midwest* (d.b.a. US Airways Express) Flight 5481. http://www.ntsb.gov/events/2003/AM5481/default.htm (last accessed Jan. 11, 2004).
14. Publications: *Aircraft accident report. Loss of pitch control during takeoff.* Air Midwest flight 5481. http://www.ntsb.gov/publictn/2004/AAR0401.htm (last accessed Jan. 11, 2004).
15. News & events: *Board meeting presentations. Air Midwest flight 5481.* http://www.ntsb.gov/events/2003/AM5481/board_meeting_presentations/presentations.htm (last accessed Jan. 11, 2004).
16. Wachter R.M., et al.: Learning from our mistakes: Quality grand rounds, a new case-based series on medical errors and patient safety (editorial). *Ann Intern Med* 136:850–852, Jun. 4, 2002.
17. Wachter R.M.: Encourage case-based discussion of medical errors. *AHA News* Feb. 9, 2004, pp. 14.
18. Piotrowski M.M., Saint S., Hinshaw D.B.: The safety case management committee: Expanding the avenues for addressing patient safety. *Jt Comm J Qual Saf* 28:296–305, Jun. 2002.
19. Allsbrook C.W., et al.: Interobserver reproducibility of Gleason grading of prostatic carcinoma. *Hum Pathol* 32:81–88, Jan. 2001.
20. Cheville J.C., Reznicek M.J., Bostwick D.G.: The focus of "atypical gland, suspicious for malignancy" in prostatic needle biopsy specimens: Incidence, histologic features, and clinical follow-up of cases diagnosed in a community practice. *Am J Clin Pathol* 108:633–640, Dec. 1997.
21. Manivel J.C.: Inconclusive results of needle biopsies of the prostate gland. *Am J Clin Pathol* 108:611–615, Dec. 1997.
22. Magi-Galluzzi C., Sanderson H., Epstein J.I.: Atypia in nonneoplastic prostate glands after radiotherapy for prostate cancer: Duration of atypia and relation to type of radiotherapy. *Am J Surg Pathol* 27:206–212, Feb. 2003.
23. Punglia R.S., et al.: Effect of verification bias on screening for prostate cancer by measurement of prostate-specific antigen. *N Engl J Med* 349:335–342, Jul. 24, 2003.
24. Kobayashi T., et al.: Detection of prostate cancer in men with prostate-specific antigen levels of 2.0 to 4.0 ng/mL equivalent to that in men with 4.1 to 10.0 ng/mL in a Japanese population. *Urology* 63:727–731, Apr. 2004.
25. Freedland S.J., et al.: Biopsy indication—A predictor of pathologic stage among men with preoperative serum PSA levels of 4.0 ng/mL or less and T1c disease. *Urology* 63:887–891, May 2004.
26. Hart E., Hazelgrove J.: Understanding the organizational context for adverse events in health services: The role of cultural censorship. *Qual Health Care* 10:257–262, Dec. 2001.
27. Christensen J.F., Levinson W., Dunn P.M.: The heart of darkness: The impact of perceived mistakes on physicians. *J Gen Int Med* 7:424–431, Jul.–Aug.1992.
28. Weeks W.B., et al.: The organizational costs of preventable medical errors. *Jt Comm J Qual Saf* 27:533–539, Oct. 2001.
29. Davidoff F.: Shame: The elephant in the room (editorial). *Qual Saf Health Care* 11:2–3, Mar. 2002.
30. When primum no nocere fails. *Lancet* 355:2007, Jun. 10, 2000.
31. Becker C.: Root-cause trouble. Court ruling in N.J. could set precedent for making JCAHO reports public. *Mod Healthc* Jun. 18, 2001, pp. 5.
32. Cook R.I.: The end of the beginning: Complexity and craftsmanship and the era of sustained work on patient safety (editorial). *Jt Comm J Qual Saf* 27:507–508, Oct. 2001.
33. Foucar E.: Error identification. *Am J Surg Pathol* 22:1–5, Jan. 1998.
34. Ramsay A.D., Gallagher P.J.: Local audit of surgical pathology. *Am J Surg Pathol* 16:476–482, May 1992.
35. Wakely S.L., et al.: Aberrant diagnoses by individual surgical pathologists. *Am J Surg Pathol* 22:77–82, Jan. 1997.
36. Ackerman A.B.: Discordance among expert pathologists in the diagnosis of melanocytic lesions. *Hum Pathol* 27:1115–1116, Nov. 1996.
37. Chapman B.: Medical mistakes. *Cap Today* 11:62–68, Jun. 1997.
38. Leape L.L.: Error in medicine. *JAMA* 272:1851–1857, Dec. 21, 1994.

Glossary of Terms

Accreditation Report In the Joint Commission accreditation process, the report resulting from the on-site assessment of an organization or network that outlines identified deficiencies in standards compliance. It also outlines the nature of the accreditation decision including enumeration of type I recommendations, the remediation of which will be monitored by the Joint Commission through focused surveys or written progress reports. The report may also include other supplemental recommendations that are designed to assist the organization or network in improving its performance.

Accreditation Watch An attribute of an organization's Joint Commission accreditation status. An organization is placed on Accreditation Watch when a reviewable sentinel event has occurred and has come to the Joint Commission's attention, and a thorough and credible root cause analysis of the sentinel event and action plan has not been completed in specified time frames. Although Accreditation Watch status is not an official accreditation category, it can be publicly disclosed by the Joint Commission.

action plan The product of the root cause analysis that identifies the strategies that an organization intends to implement to reduce the risk of similar events occurring in the future. The plan should address responsibility for implementation, oversight, pilot testing as appropriate, timelines, and strategies for measuring the effectiveness of the actions.

active failure An error that is precipitated by the commission of errors and violations. These are difficult to anticipate and have an immediate adverse affect on safety by breaching, bypassing, or disabling existing defenses.

adverse drug event (adverse drug error) Any incident in which the use of a medication (drug or biologic) at any dose, a medical device, or a special nutritional product (for example, dietary supplement, infant formula, or medical food) may have resulted in an adverse outcome in a patient.

adverse event An untoward, undesirable, and usually unanticipated event, such as death of a patient, an employee, or a visitor in a health care organization. Incidents such as patient falls or improper administration of medications are also considered adverse events, even if there is no permanent effect on the patient.

aggregate To combine standardized data and information.

aggregate data (measurement data) Measurement data collected and reported by organizations as a sum or total over a given time period (for example, monthly, quarterly), or for certain groupings (for example, health care organization level).

aggregate survey data Information on key organization performance areas and standards collected from organizations surveyed by the Joint Commission. This is combined to produce a database of information concerning the performance of the organizations during a specified time interval.

barrier analysis The study of the safeguards that can prevent or mitigate (or could have prevented or mitigated) an unwanted event or occurrence. It offers a structured way to visualize the events related to system failure or the creation of a problem.

benchmarking Continuous measurement of a process, product, or service compared to those of the toughest competitor, to those considered industry leaders, or to similar activities in the organization to find and implement ways to improve it. This is one of the foundations of both total quality management and continuous quality improvement. Internal benchmarking occurs when similar processes within the same organization are compared. Competitive benchmarking occurs when an organization's processes are compared with best practices within the industry. Functional benchmarking refers to benchmarking a similar function or process, such as scheduling, in another industry.

care The provision of accommodations, comfort, and treatment to an individual, implying responsibility for safety, including care, treatment, service, habilitation, rehabilitation, or other programs instituted by the organization for the individual served.

change analysis A study of the differences between the expected and actual performance of a process. Change analysis involves determining the root causes of an event by examining the effects of change and identifying causes.

chemical restraint The inappropriate use of a sedating psychotropic drug to manage or control behavior.

clinical pathway A treatment regime, agreed on by consensus, that includes all the elements of care, regardless of the effect on patient outcomes. It is a broader look at care and may include tests and X-rays that do not affect patient recovery. Synonyms include *clinical path* and *critical pathway*.

common-cause variation *See* variation.

complex organization An organization that provides for more than one level and type of health care service, usually in more than one type of setting. Surveying a complex organization involves the use of standards from at least two Joint Commission accreditation manuals.

complication A detrimental patient condition that arises during the process of providing health care, regardless of the setting in which the care is provided. For instance, perforation, hemorrhage, bacteremia, and adverse reactions to medication (particularly in the elderly) are four complications of colonoscopy and its associated anesthesia and sedation. A complication may prolong an inpatient's length of stay or lead to other undesirable outcomes.

coupled system A system that links two or more activities so that one process is dependent on another for completion. A system can be loosely or tightly coupled.

electronic application (e-app) for accreditation The option of applying online for accreditation through a secure password-protected Extranet site known as Jayco. An accredited organization can access Jayco six to nine months before its survey due date.

error of commission An error that occurs as a result of an action taken. Examples include a drug being administered at the wrong time, in the wrong dose, or using the wrong route; surgeries performed on the wrong side of the body; and transfusion errors involving blood cross-matched for another patient.

error of omission An error that occurs as a result of an action not taken. Examples include a delay in performing an indicated caesarean section, resulting in a fetal death; a nurse omitting a dose of a medication that should be administered; and a patient suicide that is associated with a lapse in carrying out frequent patient checks in a psychiatric unit. Errors of omission may or may not lead to adverse outcomes.

failure Lack of success, nonperformance, nonoccurrence, breaking down, or ceasing to function. In most instances, and certainly within the context of this book, failure is what is to be avoided. It takes place when a system or part of a system performs in a way that is not intended or desirable.

failure mode and effects analysis (FMEA)
A systematic way of examining a design prospectively for possible ways in which failure can occur. It assumes that no matter how knowledgeable or careful people are, errors will occur in some situations and may even be likely to occur. Synonym: *failure mode, effects, and criticality analysis (FMECA)*.

fault tree analysis A systematic way of prospectively examining a design for possible ways in which failure can occur. The analysis considers the possible direct proximate causes that could lead to the event and seeks their origins. After this is accomplished, ways to avoid these origins and causes must be identified.

flowchart (flow diagram) A pictorial summary that shows with symbols and words the steps, sequence, and relationship of the various operations involved in the performance of a function or a process.

hazard vulnerability analysis The identification of potential emergencies and the direct and indirect effects these emergencies may have on a health care organization's operations and the demand for its services.

hazardous condition Any set of circumstances (exclusive of the disease or condition for which the patient is being treated) that significantly increases the likelihood of a serious adverse outcome. *See* also latent condition.

human factors research The study of the capabilities and limitations of human performance in relation to the design of machines, jobs, and other aspects of the physical environment.

iatrogenic 1. Resulting from the professional activities of physicians, or, more broadly, from the activities of health professionals. 2. Pertaining to an illness or injury resulting from a procedure, therapy, or other element of care.

immediate cause *See* proximate cause.

incident report (occurrence report) A written report, usually completed by a nurse and forwarded to risk management personnel, that describes and provides documentation for any unusual problem, incident, or other situation that is likely to lead to undesirable effects or that varies from established policies and procedures.

indicator 1. A measure used to determine, over time, performance of functions, processes, and outcomes. 2. A statistical value that provides an indication of the condition or direction over time of performance of a defined process or achievement of a defined outcome.

individual served The terms *individual served, patient,* and *care recipient* all describe the individual, client, consumer, or resident who actually receives health care, treatment, and/or services.

Joint Commission International (JCI) JCI extends the Joint Commission's mission worldwide. Through both international consultation and accreditation, JCI helps to improve the quality and safety of patient care in many nations. JCI has extensive international experience working with public and private health care organizations and local governments in more than 40 countries.

Joint Commission on Accreditation of Healthcare Organizations An independent, not-for-profit organization dedicated to improving the quality of care in organized health care settings. Founded in 1951, its members are the American College of Physicians, the American College of Surgeons, the American Dental Association, the American Hospital Association, and the American Medical Association. The major functions of the Joint Commission include developing accreditation standards, awarding accreditation decisions, and providing education and consultation to health care organizations.

Joint Commission Resources (JCR) A not-for-profit subsidiary of the Joint Commission on Accreditation of Healthcare Organizations, JCR is dedicated to helping health care organizations improve the quality of care and achieve peak performance. JCR offers a full spectrum of resources for health care organizations including publications, education, consulting and custom education, multimedia products, and the Continuous Survey Readiness initiative, as well as international accreditation and consultation activities. JCR provides expertise on every aspect of accreditation, performance improvement and safety, and other issues health care organizations face today.

latent condition A condition that exists as a consequence of management and organizational processes and poses the greatest danger to complex systems. Latent conditions cannot be foreseen but, if detected, can be corrected before they contribute to mishaps.

licensed independent practitioner Any individual permitted by law and by an organization to provide care, treatment, and services without direction or supervision, within the scope of the individual's license and consistent with individually granted clinical privileges.

licensed practical nurse (LPN) A nurse who has completed a practical nursing program and is licensed by a state to provide routine patient care under the direction of a registered nurse or a physician. Referred to as *licensed vocational nurse (LVN)* in California and Texas.

licensure A legal right that is granted by a government agency in compliance with a statute governing an occupation (such as medicine or nursing) or the operation of an activity (such as in a long term care facility).

local trigger An intrinsic defect or atypical condition that can create failures.

malpractice Improper or unethical conduct or unreasonable lack of skill by a holder of a professional or official position; often applied to physicians, dentists, lawyers, and public officers to denote negligent or unskillful performance of duties when professional skills are obligatory.

medication Any substance, other than food or devices, that may be used on or administered to persons as an aid in the diagnosis, treatment, or prevention of disease or other abnormal condition. Synonym: *drug*.

medication error A discrepancy between what a physician orders and what is reported to occur. Types of medication errors include omission, unauthorized drug, extra dose, wrong dose, wrong dosage form, wrong rate, deteriorated drug, wrong administration technique, and wrong time. An omission medication error is the failure to give an ordered dose; a refused dose is not counted as an error if the nurse responsible for administering the dose tried, but failed, to persuade the patient to take it. Doses withheld according to written policies, such as for X-ray procedures, are not counted as omission errors. An *unauthorized drug* medication error is the administration of a dose of medication not authorized to be given to that patient. Instances of brand or therapeutic substitution are counted as unauthorized medication errors only when prohibited by organization policy. A *wrong-dose* medication error occurs when a patient receives an amount of medicine that is greater than or less than the amount ordered; the range of allowable deviation is based on each organization's definition. *See also* significant medication errors and significant adverse drug reactions; sentinel event.

near miss Used to describe any process variation that does not affect the outcome, but for which a recurrence carries a significant chance of a serious adverse outcome. Such a near miss falls within the scope of the definition of a sentinel event, but outside the scope of those sentinel events that are subject to review by the Joint Commission under its Sentinel Event Policy.

negligence Failure to use such care as a reasonably prudent and careful person would use under similar circumstances.

observation method An active method of error surveillance in which a trained observer watches the care delivery process.

occurrence report *See* incident report.

occurrence screening A system for concurrent or retrospective identification of adverse patient occurrences (APOs) through medical chart-based review according to objective screening criteria. Examples of criteria include admission for adverse results of outpatient management; readmission for complications; incomplete management of problems on previous hospitalization; or unplanned removal, injury, or repair of an organ or structure during surgery. Criteria are used organizationwide or adapted for departmental or topic-specific screening. Occurrence screening identifies about 80% to 85% of APOs. It misses APOs that are not identifiable from the medical record.

operative and other procedures Includes operative, other invasive, and noninvasive procedures that place a patient at risk. The focus is on procedures and is not meant to include medications that place a patient at risk.

outcome The result of the performance (or nonperformance) of a function(s) or process(es).

outcome database The database at the Joint Commission that stores the performance measure data and related data elements transmitted by accepted performance measurement systems.

outcome measure A measure that indicates the result of the performance (or nonperformance) of a function(s) or process(es).

Pareto chart A form of vertical bar graph that displays information in such a way that priorities for process improvement can be established. It shows the relative importance of all the data and is used to direct efforts to the largest improvement opportunity by highlighting the vital few in contrast to the many others.

Periodic Performance Review (PPR) A new form of evaluation that is conducted by the organization and focuses on patient safety and quality of care issues. The organization self-evaluates its compliance with all accreditation participation requirements, standards, and elements of performance (scoreable requirements) that are applicable to the services that the organization provides and develops a plan of action for all areas of performance identified as needing improvement.

physical restraint Any method of physically restricting an individual's freedom of movement, physical activity, or normal access to his or her body. This encompasses many physical devices, such as wrist restraints, jacket vests, and mitts.

plan-do-study-act (PDSA) cycle A four-part method for discovering and correcting assignable causes to improve the quality of processes. Synonyms: *Deming cycle, Shewhart cycle, plan-do-check-act (PDCA) cycle.*

policies and procedures The formal, approved description of how a governance, management, or clinical care process is defined, organized, and carried out.

practice guidelines Descriptive tools or standardized specification for care of a typical individual in a typical situation, developed through a formal process that incorporates the best scientific evidence of effectiveness with expert opinion. Synonyms include *clinical criteria, parameter (or practice parameter), protocol, algorithm, review criteria, preferred practice pattern, and guideline.*

practice privileges Permission to render care within well-defined limits based on an individual's professional license and his or her training, experience, competence, ability, and judgment.

practitioner Any individual who is qualified to practice a health care profession (for example, a physician or nurse). Practitioners are often required to be licensed as defined by law.

practitioner site The office of a licensed independent practitioner who is a member of the practitioner panel of a PPO or network.

preparedness activities Those activities an organization undertakes to build capacity and identify resources that may be used if an emergency occurs.

prescribing or ordering Directing the selection, preparation, or administration of medication(s).

prevention/early detection (domain) The degree to which appropriate services are provided for promotion, preservation, and restoration of health and early detection of disease.

preventive services Interventions provided by an organization to improve the health status of the populations it serves.

primary source The original source of a specific credential that can verify the accuracy of a qualification reported by an individual health care practitioner. Examples include medical school, graduate medical education program, and state medical board.

Priority Focus Process (PFP) A data-driven tool that helps focus survey activity on issues most relevant to patient safety and quality of care at the specific health care organization being surveyed.

privileging The process whereby a specific scope and content of patient care services (that is, clinical privileges) are authorized for a health care practitioner by a health care organization, based on evaluation of the individual's credentials and performance. *See also* licensed independent practitioner.

procedure 1. A series of steps taken to accomplish a desired end, as in a therapeutic, cosmetic, or surgical procedure. 2. A unit of health care, as in services and procedures.

process A goal-directed, interrelated series of actions, events, mechanisms, or steps that transform inputs into outputs.

proficiency testing 1. The assessment of technical knowledge and skills relating to certain occupations. 2. A peer comparison program used by laboratories to assess reliability of tests performed. Samples, whose precise content is unknown, are provided to laboratories for testing periodically, the results of which are compared with other laboratories who perform the same tests.

proximate cause An act or omission that naturally and directly produces a consequence. It is the superficial or obvious cause for an occurrence. Treating only the symptoms, or the proximate special cause, may lead to some short-term improvements, but does not prevent the variation from recurring.

public domain (measure) Belonging to the community at large, unprotected by copyright, and subject to appropriation by anyone.

Public Information Policy A Joint Commission policy governing the confidentiality or disclosure of information about the performance of a health care organization or network. This policy covers the Joint Commission's performance reports, information publicly disclosed on request, complaint information, aggregate performance data, data released to government agencies, and the Joint Commission's right to clarify information an accredited organization releases about its accreditation status.

quality control The performance of processes through which actual performance is measured and compared with goals, and the difference is acted on.

quality improvement An approach to the continuous study and improvement of the processes of providing health care services to meet the needs of individuals and others. Synonyms include *continuous quality* *improvement, continuous improvement, organizationwide performance improvement,* and *total quality management.*

quality of care The degree to which health services for individuals and populations increase the likelihood of desired health outcomes and are consistent with current professional knowledge. Dimensions of performance include the following: resident perspective issues; safety of the care environment; and accessibility, appropriateness, continuity, effectiveness, efficacy, efficiency, and timeliness of care.

quality reports Reports that provide consumers with relevant and useful information about the quality and safety of Joint Commission-accredited organizations. As part of its Shared Visions-New Pathways® initiative, the Joint Commission began publishing Quality Reports in July 2004.

referral The sending of an individual (1) from one clinician to another clinician or specialist, (2) from one setting or service to another, or (3) by one physician (the referring physician) to another physician(s) or other resource, either for consultation or care.

registered nurse An individual who is qualified by an approved postsecondary program or baccalaureate or higher degree in nursing and licensed by the state, commonwealth, or territory to practice professional nursing.

relevance The applicability and/or pertinence of the indicator to its users and customers. For Joint Commission purposes, face validity is subsumed in this category.

reliability The capability of an indicator to accurately and consistently identify the events it is designed to identify across multiple health care settings.

respect and caring The degree to which those providing services do so with sensitivity for an individual's needs, expectations, and individual differences, and the degree to which the individual or a designee is involved in his or her own care decisions.

restraint Any method (chemical or physical) of restricting a resident's freedom of movement (including seclusion), physical activity, or normal access to his or her body that (1) is not a usual and customary part of a medical diagnostic or treatment procedure to which the resident or his or her legal representative has consented; (2) is not indicated to treat the resident's medical condition or symptoms; or (3) does not promote the resident's independent functioning. See also *chemical restraint, physical restraint.*

risk adjustment A statistical process for reducing, removing, or clarifying the influences of confounding factors that differ among comparison groups (for example, logistic regression, stratification).

risk adjustment data elements Those data elements used to risk adjust a performance measure (such as, reduce, remove, or clarify the influences of confounding resident factors that differ among comparison groups). Such data elements may be used exclusively for risk adjustment (such as, not required to construct the numerator or denominator) or may be required for numerator or denominator construction as well as risk adjustment.

risk adjustment model The statistical algorithm that specifies the numerical values and the sequence of calculations used to risk adjust (such as, reduce or remove the influence of confounding factors) performance measures.

risk containment Immediate actions taken to safeguard patients from a repetition of an unwanted occurrence. Actions may involve removing and sequestering drug stocks from pharmacy shelves and checking or replacing oxygen supplies or specific medical devices.

risk management activities Clinical and administrative activities undertaken to identify, evaluate, and reduce the risk of injury to patients, staff, and visitors and the risk of loss to the organization itself.

risk points Specific points in a process that are susceptible to error or system breakdown. They generally result from a flaw in the initial process design, a high degree of dependence on communication, nonstandardized processes, and failure or absence of backup.

root cause A fundamental reason for the failure or inefficiency of a process.

root cause analysis A process for identifying the basic or causal factor(s) that underlie variation in performance, including the occurrence or possible occurrence of a sentinel event.

safety The degree to which the risk of an intervention (for example, use of a drug or a procedure) and risk in the care environment are reduced for a resident and other persons, including health care practitioners.

safety management A component of an organization's management of the environment of care program that maintains and improves the general safety of the care environment.

scope of care or services The activities performed by governance, managerial, clinical, or support staff.

seclusion Involuntary, solitary confinement of a person where the person is physically prevented from leaving the room.

sentinel event An unexpected occurrence involving death or serious physical or psychological injury, or the risk thereof. Serious injury specifically includes loss of limb or function. The phrase "or the risk thereof" includes any process variation for which a recurrence would carry a significant chance of a serious adverse outcome. Such events are called sentinel because they signal the need for immediate investigation and response."

services Structural divisions of an organization, its medical staff, or its licensed independent practitioner staff; also, the delivery of care.

Shared Visions-New Pathways® A Joint Commission initiative that sharpens the focus of the accreditation process on operational systems critical to the safety and quality of patient care. **Shared Visions** represents a vision that the Joint Commission has with health care organizations—as well as with health care oversight bodies and the public—to bridge what has been called a gap or chasm between the current state of health care and the potential for safer, higher quality care. **New Pathways** represents a new set of approaches or "pathways" through the accreditation process that will support fulfillment of the shared visions.

significant medication errors and significant adverse drug reactions Unintended, undesirable, and unexpected effects of prescribed medications or of medication errors that require discontinuing a medication or modifying the dose; require initial or prolonged hospitalization; result in disability; require treatment with a prescription medication; result in cognitive deterioration or impairment; are life threatening; result in death; or result in congenital anomalies. *See also* medication.

special-cause variation *See* variation.

staff Individuals, such as employees, volunteers, contractors, or temporary agency personnel, who provide services in an organization.

staff, medical or licensed independent practitioner Individuals who successfully complete a credentialing process and are granted clinical privileges by the organization.

Glossary of Terms

staffing effectiveness The number, competence, and skill mix of staff as related to the provision of needed care, treatment, and services.

standard A statement that defines the performance expectations, structures, or processes that must be substantially in place in an organization to enhance the quality of care.

standard deviation A measure of variability that indicates the spread of a set of observations around the mean.

standard of quality A generally accepted, objective standard of measurement such as a rule or guideline supported through findings from expert consensus, based on specific research and/or documentation in scientific literature, against which an individual's or organization's level of performance may be compared.

Standards Review Project A sweeping review of all the standards for all Joint Commission's accreditation programs (excluding assisted living, critical access hospitals, networks, and office-based surgery), and of the requirements for 2004 for demonstrating compliance with the standards.

Statement of Conditions™ (SOC) A proactive document that helps an organization to do a critical self-assessment of its current level of compliance and describe how to resolve any *Life Safety Code® (LSC)* deficiencies. The SOC was created to be a living, ongoing management tool that should be used in a management process that continually identifies, assesses, and resolves LSC® deficiencies.

surveillance Ongoing monitoring using methods distinguished by their practicability, uniformity, and rapidity, rather than by complete accuracy. The purpose of surveillance is to detect changes in trend or distribution to initiate investigative or control measures. Active surveillance is systematic and involves review of each case within a defined time frame. Passive surveillance is not systematic. Cases may be reported through written incident reports, verbal accounts, electronic transmission, or telephone hotlines, for example.

survey team The group of health care professionals who work together to perform a Joint Commission accreditation survey.

surveyor For purposes of Joint Commission accreditation, a physician, nurse, administrator, laboratorian, or any other health care professional who meets the Joint Commission's surveyor selection criteria, evaluates standards compliance, and provides education and consultation regarding standards compliance to surveyed organizations or networks.

system database The database at the Joint Commission that stores the profile information for each performance measurement system that has submitted their application to the Joint Commission to become a contracted performance measurement system.

tailored survey A Joint Commission survey in which standards from more than one accreditation manual are used in assessing compliance. This type of survey may include using specialist surveyors appropriate to the standards selected for survey.

tracer methodology An evaluation method in which surveyors select a patient, resident, or client and use that individual's record as a roadmap to move through an organization to assess and evaluate the organization's compliance with selected standards and the organization's systems of providing care, treatment, and services.

underlying cause The systems or process cause that allows for the proximate cause of an event to occur. Underlying causes may involve special-cause variation, common-cause variation, or both and may or may not be a root cause.

utilities management A component of an organization's management of the environment of care program designed to ensure the operational reliability, assess the special risks, and respond to failures of utility systems that support the resident care environment.

utility systems Organization systems for life support; surveillance, prevention, and control of infection; environment support; and equipment support. May include electrical distribution; emergency power; vertical and horizontal transport; heating, ventilating, and air conditioning; plumbing, boiler, and steam; piped gases; vacuum systems; or communication systems including data-exchange systems.

variation The differences in results obtained in measuring the same phenomenon more than once. The sources of variation in a process over time can be grouped into two major classes: common causes and special causes. Excessive variation frequently leads to waste and loss, such as the occurrence of undesirable patient health outcomes and increased cost of health services. Common-cause variation (also called *endogenous-cause variation* or *systemic-cause variation*) in a process is due to the process itself and is produced by interactions of variables of that process inherent in all processes, not a disturbance in the process. It can be removed only by making basic changes in the process. Special-cause variation (also called *exogenous-cause variation* or *extra-systemic cause variation*) in performance results from assignable causes. Special-cause variation is intermittent, unpredictable, and unstable. It is not inherently present in a system; rather, it arises from causes that are not part of the system as designed.

Index

A

Accreditation Committee (Joint Commission), 31, 35, 36, 37
Accreditation Watch, 31, 35, 36
Action plans. *See also* Improvement actions
  acceptability of, 31, 122
  change, creating and managing, 125, 128
  change, impact of, 119, 122
  characteristics of, 15, 118–19
  example of, 120–21
  failure reasons and remedies, 131, 132
  framework for, 23
  implementation of, 17, 120–21, 122–25
  integration of, 142
  people involved with, 139–40
  pilot testing of, 122
  purpose of, 15
  quantification of improvement, 118
  submission of, 35
Adverse events, 26. *See also* Sentinel events
  documentation tips, 42
  response to, 2
  types of, 27
Affinity diagrams
  applicability of, 148
  description of, 147
  example of, 149
  uses of, 67, 82
Agency for Healthcare Research and Quality, 1

Aggregate data indicators, 83–84
Aggregate external reference databases, 130
Aim statements, 58–59, 71
Aviation safety design characteristics, 106

B

Bar graphs, 67
Barrier analysis
  applicability of, 148
  description of, 150
  example of, 151
  uses of, 79, 94–95
Benchmarking, 130
Box plot, 148
Brainstorming
  applicability of, 148
  description of, 152
  example of, 153
  uses of, 55, 57, 67, 79, 82, 116, 125

C

Care definition, 4
Care of patients, 40
Case studies
  fall risk reduction, 175, 177–87
  wrongful surgery, 175, 189–97
Cause, 7
Cause-and-effect diagrams
  applicability of, 148
  description of, 154
  example of, 155
  uses of, 67, 79, 82, 94–95, 116, 125
Causes. *See also* Root causes

  proximate causes (see Proximate causes)
  underlying causes, 8, 93–99, 103
Change
  barriers to and solutions, 143
  creating and managing, 125, 128
  design and implementation, 85–87
  impact of, 119, 122
Change analysis, 79, 148, 156
Check sheets, 148
Clinical pathways, 124–25, 127, 130
Clinical practice guidelines, 106
Commission, errors of, 25
Common-cause variation, 8, 9–10
Communication, 40, 41–47
  frequency of, 61
  process-related failures, 99
  of results, 131, 133
Confidentiality, 37–38, 39
Contingency diagrams, 148
Continuous variable indicators, 84
Contributing factor identification, 78–82, 90–91, 100
Control charts
  applicability of, 148
  description of, 157
  example of, 158
  uses of, 78, 125, 130
Corrective actions. *See* Improvement actions
Cost-of-quality analysis, 148
Critical pathways, 124–25, 127, 130
Critical-to-quality analysis, 148
Culture of organizations, 26–27

D

Data collection, 82–85
Data tables, 125
Decision matrix, 148
Deming, W. Edwards, 123
Deployment flowchart, 148
Disclosure concerns, 39, 41–47
Documentary evidence, 65–66
Documentation of event, 40–41, 42

E

Effective-achievable matrix, 148
Elopement sentinel event, 50
   aim statement, 58–59
   improvement actions, 114–15
   information collection, 62
   literature review, 67
   reporting mechanisms, 61
   root cause analysis, minimum scope of, 16
   team membership, 53
Engineering systems design, 106
Environmental factors, 90
Environmental management issues, 96, 98–99
Equipment factors, 90, 97
Error reduction standards, 13
Errors. See Medical failures
Errors of commission, 25
Errors of omission, 25
Ethics, Rights, and Responsibilities standards, 13, 42
External databases, 130
External factors, 91, 95, 97

F

Fail-safe design, 110
Failure mode, effect, and criticality analysis (FMECA), 110–11
Failure mode and effects analysis (FMEA)
   applicability of, 148
   definition, 7
   description of, 159
   example of, 160
   purpose of, 7
   for risk reduction, 110–11
   steps in, 111
   time of use, 2
   tips, 159
   uses of, 79, 94–95, 117
Failure modes, 7
Fall risk reduction case study, 175, 177–87
Falls
   fall risk reduction case study, 175, 177–87
   root causes, 101
Fault tree analysis, 79, 94–95, 148, 161
Fishbone diagrams, 94–95, 148, 154–55
Flowcharts
   applicability of, 148
   description of, 162
   example of, 163
   uses of, 67, 78, 79, 94–95, 116, 125
FMEA. See Failure mode and effects analysis (FMEA)
FMECA (failure mode, effects, and criticality analysis), 110–11
Forced field analysis, 148
Form for reporting sentinel events, 32, 33

G

Gantt charts
   applicability of, 148
   description of, 164
   uses of, 59, 67, 86, 119
General Counsel (Joint Commission), 37
Ground rules for team meetings, 54–55
Group interviews, 65

H

Histograms, 125, 130, 148, 165–66
Human errors, 94
Human factors, 90, 97
Human resource issues, 95, 96, 98

I

Identifying the web of causation, 87
Improvement actions. See also Action plans
   barriers to implementation, 117
   defining scope and activities, 136
   defining sequence, resources, and measures, 137
   defining time frames and milestones, 138
   elopement sentinel event, 114–15
   evaluation of, 116–18, 134
   failure reasons and remedies, 131, 132
   formulation of, 111, 114–16
   locations of, 141
   medication error sentinel event, 115–16
   medication use, 111, 114
   monitoring and measurement, 146
   prioritizing, 134
   purpose of, 118
   suicide sentinel event, 114–15
   summarizing, 135
   treatment delay sentinel event, 115
Improvement goals. See Improvement actions
Improving Organization Performance standards, 11, 13, 14, 39
Indicators, 83–85
Infant abductions, 101, 109
Information
   collection of, 61–67, 73–76
   documentary evidence, 65–66

focus of collecting, 62–63
    physical evidence, 65
    protection of, 62
    recording of, 61–62
    witness statements and observations, 63–65, 73–76
Information management issues, 96, 98
Institute for Safe Medication Practices, 110
Institute of Medicine (IOM), To Err Is Human, 1
Internal comparisons, 130
Interviews, 63–65
IOM (Institute of Medicine), 1
Ishikawa diagrams, 148, 154–55
Is-is not matrix, 148

J

Johns Hopkins Children's Center, 1
Joint Commission
    Accreditation Committee, 31, 35, 36, 37
    General Counsel, 37
    Legal Affairs, Department of, 38
    Office of Quality Monitoring, 32
    Sentinel Event Advisory Group, 18
    Sentinel Event Alert, 18, 56
    Sentinel Event Database, 31, 37, 56, 58
    Sentinel Event Hotline, 15, 17, 32
    Sentinel Event Policy (see Sentinel Event Policy (Joint Commission))
    Universal Protocol for Preventing Wrong Site, Wrong Procedure, Wrong Person Surgery™, 107
    Web site, 15, 18
Joint Commission Journal on Quality and Patient Safety, 175
Joint Commission Perspectives, 27, 29, 56

K

Kolmogorov-Smirnov test, 148

L

Latent conditions, 102
Leadership
    group discussion techniques, 55
    patient safety commitment, 26–27
    process-related failures, 95, 97, 99
    of teams, 54
Leadership standards, 12, 13
"Learning to Improve Safety", 175, 189–97
Legal Affairs, Department of (Joint Commission), 37
Legal concerns, 37–38, 42, 46–47
Line graphs, 67, 125
List reduction, 148
Literature review, 66–67, 105–6
Litigation, 42, 46–47

M

Malpractice litigation, 42, 46–47
Matrix diagrams, 148
Measurement
    assessment of, 130–31
    assuring success of, 129
    choosing what to measure, 83–85
    definition, 82, 128
    development of, 128–29, 144–45
    indicators, 83–85
    performance measures, 83–85
    purpose of, 82–83, 128
    questions about, 85
    responsibility for, 129
Mechanical errors, 66
Medical failures. See also Sentinel events
    causes of, 1–2, 25
    cost of, 1
    definition of, 55–61, 69, 77–78, 88
    determining what happened, 77–78, 88
    prevalence of, 1
    response to, 2
    results of, 26
    statistics on, 1
    studying the, 61–67
Medical mistake disclosure, 42, 45–47
Medication error sentinel event, 51
    aim statement, 59
    documentary evidence, 66
    improvement actions, 115–16
    information collection, 62–63
    literature review, 67
    reporting form, 43
    reporting mechanisms, 61
    risk points, 108
    risk reduction strategies, 108
    root cause analysis, minimum scope of, 16
    root causes, 101
    team membership, 54
Medication use
    failure-preventing actions, 111, 114
    process flow diagram, 111, 112
    resolutions, 111, 115
    risk points, 111, 113
    system problems, 111, 115
Multivoting, 56, 125, 148, 167

N

National Patient Safety Goals, 18
"Near miss" events, 7, 26
Nominal group technique (NGT), 148
Normal probability plot, 148

O

Office of Quality Monitoring (Joint Commission), 32
Official Accreditation Decision Report, 36, 37
Omission, errors of, 25
Open-ended questions, 64
Operational definitions, 148
Outcome indicators, 83

P

Parameters, 130
Pareto charts
  applicability of, 148
  description of, 168
  example of, 169
  uses of, 67, 125
Patient/care recipient definition, 4
Patient falls
  case study, 175, 177–87
  root causes, 101
PDCA (plan-so-check-act) cycle, 123
PDSA (plan-do-study-act) cycle, 123–24, 125, 126, 148
Performance measures, 83–85
Performance targets, 130
Periodic Performance Review (PPR), 26
Physical evidence, 65
Physicians
  medical mistake disclosure, 42, 45–47
  performance improvement participation, 52, 54
Pie graphs, 67, 125
Plan-do-check-act (PDCA) cycle, 123
Plan-do-study-act (PDSA) cycle, 123–24, 125, 126, 148
PMI (plus, minus, interesting), 148
Practice guidelines, 130
Preliminary Denial of Accreditation, 36
Preservation of evidence, 40
Problem
  definition of, 55–61, 69, 77–78, 88
  determining what happened, 77–78, 88
  studying the, 61–67
Process design
  for medication use, 111, 112
  methods for improvement, 122–25
  safety design characteristics, 106
Process indicators, 83

Process-related failures, 78–79
  communication issues, 99
  environmental management issues, 96, 98–99
  external factors, 99
  human resource issues, 95, 96, 98
  information management issues, 96, 98
  leadership issues, 95, 97, 99
Proximate causes
  assessment factors, 80
  characteristics of, 10
  definition, 8, 78
  differentiating contributing causes, 99, 100
  environmental factors, 90
  equipment factors, 79–80, 81, 90, 97
  external factors, 91, 95, 97
  human factors, 79, 80, 90, 97
  identification of, 78–82, 85–86, 89, 93–99, 103
  procedure-related factors, 80
  tools to use, 67
  training-related factors, 81

Q

Quantification of improvement, 118
Questions, open-ended, 64

R

Rate-based indicators, 84
Redundancy, 109–10
Relations diagrams, 148
Reporting form for sentinel events, 32, 33, 43
Reporting mechanisms, 59, 61
Report of results, 131, 133
Restraint use sentinel event
  risk points, 109
  risk reduction strategies, 109
  root causes, 101, 102
Risk containment, 40

Risk points, 57, 70, 107–9
  medication error sentinel event, 108
  medication use, 111, 113
  restraint use sentinel event, 109
  wrongful surgery case study, 107
Risk-prone systems, 70
Risk reduction strategies
  fail-safe design, 110
  failure mode and effects analysis (FMEA) (see Failure mode and effects analysis (FMEA))
  identification of, 110
  infant abductions, 109
  literature review, 105–6
  medication error sentinel event, 108
  planning, 106
  redundancy, 109–10
  restraint use sentinel event, 109
  suicide sentinel event, 109
  systems approach to, 106–7
  wrongful surgery case study, 107
The Root Cause Analysis Handbook, 63
Root cause analysis
  acceptability of, 31
  acceptable, characteristics of, 14
  benefits of, 10–14
  credible, characteristics of, 15
  definition, 7
  framework for, 20–23
  identifying the web of causation, 87
  matrix, 16
  minimum scope of, 15, 16
  purpose of, 7, 15, 17
  resources needed for, 8
  steps in, 60
  submission of, 35
  thorough, characteristics of, 14
  time of use, 2, 7

Root causes
   categories of, 95–99
   characteristics of, 10
   differentiating contributing causes, 99, 100
   identification of, 93–99, 101–2
   number to identify, 99, 101–2
Run charts
   applicability of, 148
   description of, 170
   example of, 170
   uses of, 125, 130

S

Safety and health care error reduction standards, 13
Safety design characteristics, 106
Samples. See Worksheets and samples
Scatter diagrams (scattergram)
   applicability of, 148
   description of, 171
   example of, 172
   uses of, 67, 125
Scientific method, 116
Sentinel Event Advisory Group (Joint Commission), 18
Sentinel Event Alert (Joint Commission), 18, 56
Sentinel Event Database (Joint Commission), 31, 37, 56, 58
Sentinel Event Hotline (Joint Commission), 15, 17, 32
Sentinel event indicators, 83–84
Sentinel event policy
   communication, 41–47
   confidentiality, 39
   development of, 38–40, 41
   disclosure concerns, 39, 41–47
   discoverability concerns, 39
   documentation of event, 40–41
   notification checklist, 41, 44
   reporting form, 32, 33, 43
   response strategies, 40

Sentinel Event Policy (Joint Commission), 14
   Accreditation Watch, 34, 35
   action plan, acceptability of, 31
   action plan submission, 35
   clarification of questions on, 15
   confidentiality, 37–38
   disclosable information, 34
   document handling, 37
   failure to report, 34
   follow-up activities, 37
   goals of, 29
   information on, 18
   Joint Commission's response to sentinel events, 36
   nonreviewable events, 26, 27, 31, 32
   on-site review, 34, 35
   process flow, 27–29
   reportable events, 26
   reporting form, 32, 33
   reporting of, 30–31, 32–33, 35–36
   reporting of, reasons for, 31–32
   reviewable events, 26, 27, 29, 30, 58
   reviewable events, response to, 34–35
   root cause analysis, acceptability of, 31
   root cause analysis submission, 35
   survey process, 29
Sentinel events. See also Sentinel Event Policy (Joint Commission)
   causes of, 9, 25–26, 56, 57
   challenges from, 8
   definition, 7, 25, 39
   example of, 50–51
   indicators, 83–84
   Joint Commission requirements, 10–14
   prevalence of, 8
   reporting of, 18
   response to, 2, 26–27
   review process, 26

   root cause analysis, minimum scope of, 15, 16
   root cause analysis use, 10
   statistics on, 18
   types of, 15
   Web site information, 18
   work plan for investigation, 57–59, 60
Shewart, Walter, 123
Special-cause variation, 7, 8–10, 78, 94
Standards
   Ethics, Rights, and Responsibilities, 13, 42
   Improving Organization Performance, 11, 13, 14, 39
   Leadership, 12, 13–14
   safety and health care error reduction, 13
Storyboards, 148
Stratification, 148
Suicide sentinel event, 50
   aim statement, 58
   change design and implementation, 85–86
   documentary evidence, 66
   improvement actions, 114–15
   information collection, 62
   literature review, 67
   reporting mechanisms, 61
   risk reduction strategies, 109
   root cause analysis, minimum scope of, 16
   root causes, 101
   team membership, 53
Survey process, 29
Systems approach, 106–7

T

Targets, performance, 130
Team meeting ground rules, 54–55
Team organization, 49, 51–55, 130
   group discussion techniques, 55
   team composition, 52–54, 68

team leadership, 54
team size, 54
Telephone interviews, 65
Timelines, 67, 78, 148, 173
To Err Is Human (IOM), 1
Tools and techniques
    affinity diagrams, 67, 82, 147, 148, 149
    bar graphs, 67
    barrier analysis, 79, 94–95, 148, 150–51
    box plot, 148
    brainstorming (see Brainstorming)
    cause-and-effect diagrams (see Cause-and-effect diagrams)
    change analysis, 79, 148, 156
    check sheets, 148
    contingency diagrams, 148
    control charts (see Control charts)
    cost-of-quality analysis, 148
    critical-to-quality analysis, 148
    data tables, 125
    decision matrix, 148
    deployment flowchart, 148
    effective-achievable matrix, 148
    failure mode and effects analysis (see Failure mode and effects analysis (FMEA))
    fault tree analysis, 79, 94–95, 148, 161
    fishbone diagrams, 94–95, 148, 154–55
    flowcharts (see Flowcharts)
    forced field analysis, 148
    Gantt charts (see Gantt charts)
    histograms, 125, 130, 148, 165–66
    Ishikawa diagrams, 148, 154–55
    is-is not matrix, 148
    Kolmogorov-Smirnov tests, 148
    line graphs, 67, 125
    list reduction, 148
    matrix diagrams, 148
    multivoting, 56, 125, 148, 167
    nominal group technique (NGT), 148
    normal probability plot, 148
    operational definitions, 148
    Pareto charts (see Pareto charts)
    PDSA (plan-do-study-act) cycle, 123–24, 125, 126, 148
    pie graphs, 67, 125
    plan-do-study-act (PDSA) cycle, 123–24, 125, 126, 148
    PMI (plus, minus, interesting), 148
    relations diagrams, 148
    run charts (see Run charts)
    scatter diagrams (scattergram), 67, 125, 148, 171–72
    storyboards, 148
    stratification, 148
    timelines, 67, 78, 148, 173
    top-down flowcharts, 148
    why-why not diagrams, 148
    work-flow diagrams, 148
Top-down flowcharts, 148
Treatment delay sentinel event, 50
    aim statement, 59
    improvement actions, 115
    information collection, 62
    literature review, 67
    reporting mechanisms, 61
    root cause analysis, minimum scope of, 16
    root causes, 101
    team membership, 53–54

U

Underlying causes, 8, 93–99, 103
Universal Protocol for Preventing Wrong Site, Wrong Procedure, Wrong Person Surgery™, 107
U.S. Department of Veterans Affairs (VA), 175
"Using Aggregate Root Cause Analysis to Reduce Falls and Related Injuries", 175, 177–87

V

VA National Center for Patient Safety, 110
Variation, 8–10
Veterans Affairs Ann Arbor Healthcare System (VAAAHS), 175, 189–97

W

Web of causation, 87
Web sites
    General Counsel (Joint Commission), 37
    Joint Commission, 15, 18
    Joint Commission Perspectives, 29
    Legal Affairs, Department of (Joint Commission), 37
    Office of Quality Monitoring (Joint Commission), 32
    Sentinel Event Hotline, 17
    sentinel events information, 18
Why-why diagram, 148
Witness statements and observations, 63–65, 73–76
Work-flow diagram, 148
Work plan for investigation, 57–59, 60, 72
Worksheets and samples
    aim statement, 71
    change barriers and solutions, 143
    composing the team, 68
    defining the problem, 69, 88
    evaluating target goals, 146
    factors close to the event identification, 90–91
    framework for a root cause analysis and action plan, 20–23
    improvement actions, location of, 141
    improvement actions, prioritizing, 134
    improvement actions, scope and activities, 136

improvement actions, summarizing, 135
improvement goals, sequence, resources, and measures, 137
improvement goals time frames and milestones, 138
information gathering, 73–76
integrating the improvement plan, 142
involving the right people, 139–40
measurement plan design, 144–45
medication error occurrence report, 43
planning, preliminary, 72
proximate causes identification, 86, 89
risk-prone systems, 70
root cause analysis, steps in, 60
root cause and contributing cause differentiation, 100
self-reported sentinel event, 33
sentinel event notification checklist, 44
underlying causes identification, 103

Wrongful surgery case study, 175, 189–97
  change design and implementation, 86
  risk points, 107
  risk reduction strategies, 107
  root causes, 101